Workbook for
Hartman's Nursing Assistant Care
Long-Term Care and Home Care

By Hartman Publishing, Inc.

THIRD EDITION

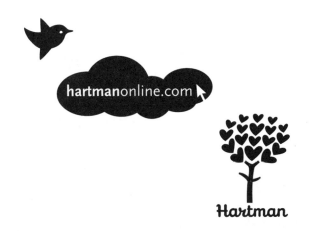

hartmanonline.com

Hartman

Credits

Managing Editor
Susan Alvare Hedman

Cover Designer
Kirsten Browne

Production
Tracy Kopsachilis

Proofreaders
Sara Alexander
Sapna Desai
Joanna Owusu

Copyright Information

© 2019 by Hartman Publishing, Inc.
1313 Iron Avenue SW
Albuquerque, New Mexico 87102
(505) 291-1274
web: hartmanonline.com
e-mail: orders@hartmanonline.com
Twitter: @HartmanPub

ISBN 978-1-60425-101-2

PRINTED IN THE USA

Third Printing, 2021

Notice to Readers

Though the guidelines and procedures contained in this text are based on consultations with healthcare professionals, they should not be considered absolute recommendations. The instructor and readers should follow employer, local, state, and federal guidelines concerning healthcare practices. These guidelines change, and it is the reader's responsibility to be aware of these changes and of the policies and procedures of his or her healthcare facility.

The publisher, author, editors, and reviewers cannot accept any responsibility for errors or omissions or for any consequences from application of the information in this book and make no warranty, express or implied, with respect to the contents of the book. The publisher does not warrant or guarantee any of the products described herein or perform any analysis in connection with any of the product information contained herein.

Gender Usage

This workbook uses gender pronouns interchangeably to denote healthcare team members and residents.

Please do not copy our workbook. Report violations to legal@hartmanonline.com.

Table of Contents

Preface v

1 Understanding Healthcare Settings 1

2 The Nursing Assistant and the Care Team 5

3 Legal and Ethical Issues 11

4 Communication and Cultural Diversity 17

5 Infection Prevention and Control 27

6 Safety and Body Mechanics 35

7 Emergency Care and Disaster Preparation 41

8 Human Needs and Human Development 45

9 The Healthy Human Body 53

10 Positioning, Transfers, and Ambulation 61

11 Admitting, Transferring, and Discharging 65

12 The Resident's Unit 69

13 Personal Care Skills 73

14 Basic Nursing Skills 79

15 Nutrition and Hydration 85

16 Urinary Elimination 95

17 Bowel Elimination 99

18 Common Chronic and Acute Conditions 103

19 Confusion, Dementia, and Alzheimer's Disease 115

20 Mental Health and Mental Illness 123

21 Rehabilitation and Restorative Care 127

22 Special Care Skills 131

23 Dying, Death, and Hospice 135

24 Introduction to Home Care 141

25 Infection Prevention and Safety in the Home 145

26 Medications in Home Care 149

27 New Mothers, Infants, and Children 153

28 Meal Planning, Shopping, Preparation, and Storage .. 159

29 The Clean, Safe, and Healthy Home Environment ... 163

30 Managing Time, Energy, and Money in the Home ... 169

31 Caring for Your Career and Yourself 171

Procedure Checklists 177

Practice Exam 229

iv

Preface

Welcome to the *Workbook for Nursing Assistant Care: Long-Term Care and Home Care*! This workbook is designed to help you review what you have learned from reading your textbook. For this reason, the workbook is organized around learning objectives, just like the textbook and even your instructor's teaching material.

These learning objectives work as a built-in study guide. After completing the exercises for each learning objective in the workbook, ask yourself if you can DO what that learning objective describes.

If you can, move on to the next learning objective. If you cannot, just go back to the textbook, reread that learning objective, and try again.

We have provided procedure checklists close to the end of the workbook. There is also a practice test for the certification exam. The answers to the workbook exercises are in your instructor's teaching guide.

Happy Learning!

1

Understanding Healthcare Settings

1. Discuss the structure of the healthcare system and describe ways it is changing

Multiple Choice
Circle the letter of the answer that best completes the statement or answers the question.

1. Another name for a long-term care facility is
   (A) Skilled nursing facility
   (B) Home healthcare facility
   (C) Assisted living facility
   (D) Adult day services facility

2. Assisted living facilities are initially for
   (A) People who need 24-hour skilled care
   (B) People who need some help with daily care
   (C) People who will die within six months
   (D) People who need acute care

3. Which of the following statements is true of adult day services?
   (A) This type of care is for people who need to live in the facility where care is provided.
   (B) This type of care is for people who need some assistance and supervision during certain hours.
   (C) Most people who need adult day services are seriously ill or disabled.
   (D) Many types of outpatient surgeries are performed at adult day services centers.

4. Care given by specialists to restore or improve function after an illness or injury is called
   (A) Acute care
   (B) Subacute care
   (C) Rehabilitation
   (D) Hospice care

5. Care given to people who have approximately six months or less to live is called
   (A) Acute care
   (B) Subacute care
   (C) Rehabilitative care
   (D) Hospice care

6. Home health aides
   (A) May clean or shop for groceries
   (B) Have no contact with the client's family and/or friends
   (C) Do not have any supervision
   (D) Are not allowed to provide personal care

7. People who live in a long-term care facility are usually called _____ because it is where they live for the duration of their stay.
   (A) Patients
   (B) Healthcare providers
   (C) Regulators
   (D) Residents

8. Most conditions in long-term care are chronic. This means that
   (A) The conditions require immediate treatment at a hospital.
   (B) The conditions last a long time.
   (C) The conditions last a short time.
   (D) The conditions will usually cause death within three months.

Matching

For each of the following definitions, write the letter of the correct definition from the list below. Use each letter only once.

9. ____ Facilities

10. ____ HMOs (health maintenance organizations)

11. ____ Managed care

12. ____ Payers

13. ____ PPOs (preferred provider organizations)

14. ____ Providers

(A) Cost-control strategies for health care

(B) People or organizations that provide health care

(C) Places where health care is delivered or administered

(D) A health plan that states that customers must use a particular doctor or group of doctors

(E) People or organizations paying for health-care services

(F) A network of providers that contract to provide health services to a group of people

2. Describe a typical long-term care facility

True or False

Mark each statement with either a T for true or an F for false.

1. ____ Long-term care facilities may offer assisted living, subacute care, or specialized care.

2. ____ Facilities that offer specialized care must have specially trained employees.

3. ____ Nonprofit organizations cannot own long-term care facilities.

3. Describe residents who live in long-term care facilities

Multiple Choice

1. What is the most important thing for a nursing assistant to know about the residents in her care?
   (A) Whether or not residents have family close by
   (B) How long residents have been in the facility
   (C) That each resident is an individual with his own abilities and needs
   (D) When residents normally have visitors

2. More than half of residents in long-term care facilities are
   (A) Younger than 50 years old
   (B) Female
   (C) Male
   (D) Developmentally disabled children

3. In general, residents who stay at a facility for more than six months
   (A) Need 24-hour care
   (B) Have caregivers available to them in the community
   (C) Are suffering from a terminal illness
   (D) Are likely to return to live in the community

Short Answer

4. Why is it important for nursing assistants to care for each resident as a whole person instead of treating only his or her disorders and disabilities?

_____

_____

_____

_____

_____

_____

_____

_____

_____

_____

4. Explain policies and procedures

True or False

1. ____ A policy is a course of action to be followed. For example, all healthcare information must remain confidential.

2. ____ Facilities will have procedures for reporting information about residents.

3. ____ It is all right to perform tasks not listed in the job description if they are very simple.

4. ____ Changes in residents' conditions should be reported to the nurse.

5. ____ Each step in a procedure is important and must be strictly followed.

5. Describe the long-term care survey process

Multiple Choice

1. What is the purpose of surveys in long-term care facilities?
   (A) To count the number of residents
   (B) To refine the care-planning process
   (C) To study how well residents are cared for
   (D) To help the facility decide appropriate visiting hours

2. If a surveyor asks a nursing assistant (NA) a question, and the NA does not know the answer, what would be her best response?
   (A) The NA should try to guess the correct answer.
   (B) The NA should offer information on another topic.
   (C) The NA should try to tell the surveyor what she thinks he wants to hear.
   (D) The NA should admit that she does not know and should find out the answer.

3. Which of the following statements is true of the Joint Commission?
   (A) Long-term care facilities are required by federal law to participate in the Joint Commission's surveys.
   (B) State surveys are the same as the Joint Commission's surveys.
   (C) The goal of the Joint Commission's survey process is to improve safety and quality of care.
   (D) The Joint Commission makes decisions relating to Medicaid eligibility.

6. Explain Medicare and Medicaid

Short Answer

1. List two groups of people who qualify for Medicare.

   _____

   _____

   _____

   _____

   _____

2. List the four parts of Medicare and what each helps pay for.

   _____

   _____

   _____

   _____

   _____

   _____

   _____

   _____

3. How is eligibility for Medicaid determined?

   _____

   _____

   _____

7. Discuss the terms *culture change* and *person-centered care*

Short Answer

1. List four examples of how you think elderly people living in care facilities can benefit from person-directed care.

_____

_____

_____

_____

_____

_____

_____

_____

_____

_____

_____

_____

_____

_____

_____

_____

_____

_____

_____

_____

_____

_____

2

The Nursing Assistant and the Care Team

1. Identify the members of the care team and describe how the care team works together to provide care

Matching
Use each letter only once.

1. ____ Activities Director

2. ____ Licensed Practical Nurse (LPN) or Licensed Vocational Nurse (LVN)

3. ____ Medical Social Worker (MSW)

4. ____ Nursing Assistant (NA or CNA)

5. ____ Occupational Therapist (OT)

6. ____ Physical Therapist (PT or DPT)

7. ____ Physician or Doctor (MD or DO)

8. ____ Registered Dietitian (RDT)

9. ____ Registered Nurse (RN)

10. ____ Resident

11. ____ Speech-Language Pathologist (SLP)

(A) Performs assigned tasks, such as measuring vital signs, providing personal care, and reporting observations to other care team members

(B) Diagnoses disease or disability and prescribes treatment

(C) Licensed professional who has completed one to two years of education and is able to administer medications and give treatments

(D) Person whose condition, goals, priorities, treatment, and progress are what the care team revolves around

(E) Develops a treatment plan to increase movement, improve circulation, promote healing, reduce pain, prevent disability, and regain mobility

(F) Identifies communication disorders and creates a care plan, as well as teaches exercises to help the resident improve or overcome speech problems

(G) Helps residents learn to adapt to disabilities by training them to perform activities of daily living and other activities

(H) Assesses a resident's nutritional status and develops a treatment plan that may include creating special diets

(I) Helps residents get support services, such as counseling

(J) Coordinates, manages, and provides skilled nursing care, as well as supervises nursing assistants' daily care of residents

(K) Plans activities to help residents socialize and stay mentally and physically active

2. Explain the nursing assistant's role

Short Answer

1. What are three tasks that nursing assistants are not allowed to perform?

_____

_____

_____

_____

_____

_____

2. What is one reason that observing and reporting changes in a resident's condition is important?

_____
_____
_____
_____

3. If a nursing assistant sees a resident who is not on his assignment sheet but who needs help, what should the NA do?

_____
_____
_____
_____

3. Explain professionalism and list examples of professional behavior

Short Answer
Mark each of the following items with a P for professional behavior or a U for unprofessional behavior.

1. _____ Being on time for work

2. _____ Being neatly dressed and groomed

3. _____ Doing tasks that have not been assigned if the resident requests them

4. _____ Keeping resident information confidential

5. _____ Telling a resident about a bad date that the nursing assistant had over the weekend

6. _____ Explaining care before providing it

7. _____ Accepting a birthday gift from a resident

8. _____ Providing person-centered care

9. _____ Asking questions when not sure of something

10. _____ Calling a favorite resident *Sweetie*

11. _____ Being a positive role model

Matching
Use each letter only once.

12. _____ Compassionate

13. _____ Conscientious

14. _____ Dependable

15. _____ Empathetic

16. _____ Honest

17. _____ Patient

18. _____ Respectful

19. _____ Sympathetic

20. _____ Tactful

21. _____ Tolerant

22. _____ Unprejudiced

(A) Being caring, concerned, considerate, empathetic, and understanding

(B) Giving the same quality of care regardless of age, gender, sexual orientation, religion, race, ethnicity, or condition

(C) Being guided by a sense of right and wrong

(D) Valuing other people's individuality and treating others politely and kindly

(E) Showing sensitivity and having a sense of what is appropriate when dealing with others

(F) Being truthful

(G) Getting to work on time and doing assigned tasks skillfully

(H) Respecting others' beliefs and practices and not judging others

(I) Identifying with the feelings of others

(J) Sharing in the feelings and difficulties of others

(K) Not losing one's temper easily, not acting irritated or annoyed, not rushing residents

4. Describe proper personal grooming habits

Multiple Choice

1. Why is proper grooming important for nursing assistants (NAs)?
   (A) Proper grooming helps NAs get to work on time.
   (B) Proper grooming improves the accuracy of documentation.
   (C) Proper grooming affects how confident residents feel about the care NAs give.
   (D) Proper grooming helps NAs to be more compassionate.

2. How often should a nursing assistant bathe?
   (A) Once a week
   (B) Twice a week
   (C) Every other day
   (D) Every day

3. Which of the following items should nursing assistants not use before going to work?
   (A) Deodorant
   (B) Toothpaste
   (C) Perfume
   (D) Shampoo

4. Hair should always be
   (A) Hanging loosely around the face
   (B) Brushed or combed
   (C) Dyed
   (D) Cut short

5. Which of the following would be a good type of clothing for a nursing assistant to wear to work?
   (A) Tight shirt with baggy pants
   (B) See-through blouse and capri pants
   (C) Clean, ironed uniform
   (D) T-shirt and short skirt

6. Which of the following would be the best choice for a nursing assistant to wear to work?
   (A) Ring
   (B) Watch
   (C) Bangle bracelets
   (D) Cuff links

7. Why should artificial nails not be worn to work?
   (A) They may not match the uniform.
   (B) Confused residents may want to eat them.
   (C) They make it more difficult to chart observations.
   (D) They harbor bacteria.

5. Explain the chain of command and scope of practice

Multiple Choice

1. Which of the following statements is true of the chain of command?
   (A) It describes the line of authority.
   (B) It is the same as the care team.
   (C) It details the survey process for each facility.
   (D) Nursing assistants are at the top of the chain of command.

2. Liability is a legal term that means
   (A) The line of authority in a facility
   (B) Ignoring a resident's call light
   (C) Someone can be held responsible for harming someone else
   (D) A task that a person is not trained for

3. Why should a nursing assistant not perform tasks that are not assigned to him?
   (A) The NA may be assigned more work if he performs additional tasks.
   (B) The NA may put himself or a resident in danger.
   (C) The NA may need to pay for additional training.
   (D) The NA may have to arrive at work earlier.

Short Answer

4. Define *scope of practice*.

_____

_____

_____

_____

_____

_____

_____

_____

_____

5. List three tasks that are said to be outside the scope of practice of a nursing assistant.

_____

_____

_____

_____

_____

_____

_____

_____

_____

6. Discuss the resident care plan and explain its purpose

True or False

1. _____ The purpose of the care plan is to give suggestions for care, which the nursing assistant can customize for each resident.

2. _____ Nursing assistants should not perform activities that are not listed on the care plan.

3. _____ Care planning only involves the doctor's diagnosis; it does not involve the resident's input or expectations.

4. _____ Sometimes even simple observations that nursing assistants make about residents are very important.

7. Describe the nursing process

Multiple Choice

1. The assessment step of the nursing process involves
   (A) Getting information about the resident and reviewing this information
   (B) Identifying health problems and resident needs
   (C) Setting goals and creating a care plan
   (D) Deciding if goals were met

2. The diagnosis step of the nursing process involves
   (A) Getting information about the resident and reviewing this information
   (B) Identifying health problems and resident needs
   (C) Deciding if goals were met
   (D) Putting the care plan into action

3. The planning step of the nursing process involves
   (A) Getting information about the resident and reviewing this information
   (B) Identifying health problems and resident needs
   (C) Putting the care plan into action
   (D) Setting goals and creating a care plan

4. The implementation step of the nursing process involves
   (A) Identifying health problems and resident needs
   (B) Putting the care plan into action
   (C) Setting goals and creating a care plan
   (D) Deciding if goals were met

5. The evaluation step of the nursing process involves
   (A) Identifying health problems and resident needs
   (B) Deciding if goals were met
   (C) Putting the care plan into action
   (D) Setting goals and creating a care plan

6. The goal of the nursing process is to
(A) Train the care team staff to work with the resident
(B) Protect the facility from liability
(C) Plan and evaluate the resident's care needs
(D) Keep resident information confidential

_____

_____

_____

_____

_____

_____

8. Describe *The Five Rights of Delegation*

Fill in the Blank

Questions to ask before delegating a task include the following:

1. Is there a match between the resident's _____ and the NA's skills, _____, and experience?

2. What is the level of resident _____?

3. Can the nurse give appropriate direction and _____?

4. Is the nurse available to give _____, support, and help?

Questions to ask before accepting a task include the following:

5. Do I have all the _____ I need to do this job?

6. Do I have the necessary _____ for the task?

7. Do I have the needed supplies, _____, and other support?

8. Do I know how to reach my _____?

9. Demonstrate how to manage time and assignments

Short Answer

1. List five guidelines for managing time.

_____

_____

_____

Name: _____

3

Legal and Ethical Issues

1. Define the terms *law* and *ethics* and list examples of legal and ethical behavior

Short Answer

For each of the following examples, decide whether the issue is a legal issue or an ethical issue. Write L for legal or E for ethical.

1. _____ Dorothy, a nursing assistant, makes fun of the way one of her residents speaks English when she is at home with her husband.

2. _____ Dennis, a nursing assistant, takes a book from a resident with dementia to give to a friend.

3. _____ Lisa is ten minutes late coming in for work on Monday. Her supervisor does not notice and Lisa does not tell her.

4. _____ Paula is having trouble completing her procedures on time. She is afraid of losing her job, so she makes up a blood pressure reading on a resident's chart.

Read each of the following scenarios and answer the questions.

5. Sarah, a nursing assistant, is out shopping with her friends. One of them asks her if she likes her job, and she responds enthusiastically. She proceeds to relate to them that her resident, Mrs. Daly, has Alzheimer's disease and has to be reminded of her name several times a day, as she is apt to forget it.

Did Sarah behave in a legal and ethical manner? Why or why not?

_____

_____

_____

_____

6. Caroyl, a nursing assistant, finishes her duties for the day and is about to leave. One of her residents, Mr. Leach, tells her how pleased he is with her work. He says that she is the first NA that has made him feel so comfortable and well taken care of. He gives her a little box of candy and says it is for all the hard work she has done. Caroyl initially refuses, but after he insists, she takes it from him, thanking him.

Did Caroyl behave in a legal and ethical manner? Why or why not?

_____

_____

_____

_____

7. Mark, a nursing assistant, has been working at a facility for almost a year. One of his residents, Mrs. Hedman, has family visiting her from out of state. Mark meets her daughter, Susan, for the first time. During the course of conversation, Susan asks Mark to come have a drink with her so they can talk about her mother's case in a more relaxed environment. Mark tells her that he can go out for a short while. They arrange to meet.

Did Mark behave in a legal and ethical manner? Why or why not?

_____

_____

Legal and Ethical Issues

_____
_____
_____
_____
_____
_____
_____

2. Explain the Omnibus Budget Reconciliation Act (OBRA)

Multiple Choice

1. The Omnibus Budget Reconciliation Act (OBRA) sets minimum standards for
   (A) Facility cleanliness
   (B) Resident budget management
   (C) Nursing assistant training
   (D) Facility spending

2. According to OBRA, nursing assistants must complete at least ___ hours of training and pass a competency evaluation before they can be employed.
   (A) 100
   (B) 250
   (C) 50
   (D) 75

3. Which of the following topics is required by OBRA to be covered during nursing assistant (NA) training?
   (A) Healthcare coverage for nursing assistants
   (B) Promoting residents' legal rights
   (C) Meal preparation for residents
   (D) Hours and days that nursing assistants are available to work

4. The Minimum Data Set (MDS) is a form for
   (A) Listing staff requirements for each long-term care facility
   (B) Detailing the minimum services that long-term care facilities must provide
   (C) Describing the number of hours of training that nursing assistants must complete each year
   (D) Assessing residents and solving resident problems

5. How often must an MDS be completed for each resident?
   (A) Any time there is a major change in a resident's condition
   (B) Every six months
   (C) Never, unless a serious problem exists
   (D) Every two years

3. Explain Residents' Rights and discuss why they are important

Multiple Choice
Read each of the following scenarios. Decide which of the Residents' Rights is being violated in each, and circle the correct letter.

1. Mrs. Perkins is a resident who is visually impaired. She is nearsighted and has misplaced her glasses many times. She gets upset during eye examinations, so the staff at her facility often allow her to go without glasses for a few weeks before having them replaced. Which Residents' Right is being violated?
   (A) Services and activities to maintain a high level of wellness
   (B) The right to complain
   (C) The right to make independent choices
   (D) The right to privacy and confidentiality

2. Mr. Gallerano has a stomach ulcer that gives him minor pain. He has medication for it, but he says it makes him nauseated and he does not want to take it. Lila, a nursing assistant, tells him that he may not have his dinner until he takes the medication. Which Residents' Right is being violated?
   (A) The right to be fully informed about rights and services
   (B) The right to participate in their own care
   (C) The right to security of possessions
   (D) The right to privacy and confidentiality

3. Ms. Mayes, a resident with severe arthritis, has a blue sweater that she loves to wear. The buttons are very tiny, and she cannot button them herself. Jim, a nursing assistant, tells her that she cannot wear the sweater today because it takes him too long to help her into it. Which Residents' Right is being violated?
(A) The right to make independent choices
(B) The right to participate in their own care
(C) The right to be fully informed about rights and services
(D) The right to privacy and confidentiality

4. Amy is a nursing assistant at Sweetwater Retirement Home. Every night when she goes home, she tells her family touching stories about the residents with whom she works. Which Residents' Right is being violated?
(A) The right to be fully informed about rights and services
(B) The right to participate in their own care
(C) The right to make independent choices
(D) The right to privacy and confidentiality

5. Laura, a nursing assistant at Great Oak Nursing Home, is running behind with her work for the evening. She is helping Mr. Young, a resident with Alzheimer's disease, with his dinner. She is getting frustrated with him because he keeps taking the fork out of her hand and dropping it on the floor. Finally, she slaps his hand to get him to stop. Which Residents' Right is being violated?
(A) The right to security of possessions
(B) The right to complain
(C) The right to dignity, respect, and freedom
(D) The right to visits

6. Mrs. Hart is a resident with dementia at Longmeadow Retirement Home. She is usually unresponsive to her surroundings. James, a nursing assistant, notices a pretty bracelet on her dresser. He borrows it for his wife to wear to a formal dinner party, knowing that Mrs. Hart will not notice. Which Residents' Right is being violated?
(A) The right to security of possessions
(B) The right to complain
(C) The right to make independent choices
(D) The right to visits

7. Ms. Land, an elderly resident, gets into a loud argument with another resident during a card game. When her daughter comes to see her later that day, Anne, an NA, tells her that Ms. Land is in a bad mood and cannot see anyone. Which Residents' Right is being violated?
(A) The right to security of possessions
(B) Transfer and discharge rights
(C) The right to make independent choices
(D) The right to visits

8. During dinner, Pete, a nursing assistant, spills hot soup on a resident's arm. He tells her that she had better not tell anyone about it or he will be very angry at her. Which Residents' Right is being violated?
(A) The right to security of possessions
(B) Transfer and discharge rights
(C) The right to visits
(D) The right to complain

4. Discuss abuse and neglect and explain how to report abuse and neglect

Matching
Use each letter only once.

1. _____ Abuse

2. _____ Active neglect

3. _____ Assault

4. _____ Battery

5. _____ Domestic violence

6. _____ False imprisonment

7. _____ Financial abuse

8. _____ Involuntary seclusion

9. _____ Malpractice

10. _____ Neglect

11. _____ Negligence

12. _____ Passive neglect

13. _____ Physical abuse

14. _____ Psychological abuse

15. _____ Sexual abuse

Name: _____

16. _____ Sexual harassment

17. _____ Substance abuse

18. _____ Verbal abuse

19. _____ Workplace violence

(A) Actions, or failure to act or provide proper care, resulting in unintended injury to a person

(B) The repeated use of legal or illegal drugs, cigarettes, or alcohol in a way that harms oneself or others

(C) Any unwelcome sexual advance or behavior that creates an intimidating, hostile, or offensive work environment

(D) The purposeful failure to give needed care, resulting in harm to a person

(E) The separation of a person from others against the person's will

(F) Verbal, physical, or sexual abuse of staff by other staff members or residents

(G) The intentional touching of a person without his or her consent

(H) A threat resulting in a person feeling fearful that he or she will be harmed

(I) The improper or illegal use of a person's money, possessions, property, or other assets

(J) The forcing of a person to perform or participate in sexual acts

(K) The use of spoken or written words, pictures, or gestures that threaten, embarrass, or insult a person

(L) Emotional harm caused by threatening, scaring, humiliating, intimidating, isolating, or insulting a person, or by treating him or her like a child

(M) Physical, sexual, or emotional abuse by spouses, intimate partners, or family members

(N) Purposeful mistreatment that causes physical, mental, or emotional pain or injury to someone

(O) Any treatment, intentional or unintentional, that causes harm to a person's body—includes slapping, bruising, cutting, burning, physically restraining, pushing, shoving, and rough handling

(P) The unintentional failure to provide needed care, resulting in physical, mental, or emotional harm to a person

(Q) Unlawful restraint that affects a person's freedom of movement

(R) Injury caused by professional misconduct through negligence, carelessness, or lack of skill

(S) The failure to provide needed care that results in physical, mental, or emotional harm to a person

Short Answer

20. What are mandated reporters?

_____

_____

_____

_____

_____

_____

_____

21. If a resident wants to make a complaint of abuse, what must a nursing assistant do?

_____

_____

_____

_____

_____

_____

_____

_____

5. List examples of behavior supporting and promoting Residents' Rights

Multiple Choice

1. When performing a procedure on a resident, the nursing assistant (NA) should
   (A) Try to distract the resident so she will not know what the NA is doing
   (B) Explain the procedure fully before performing it
   (C) Wait until the resident is reading before starting the procedure
   (D) Talk to the resident's roommate so the resident does not become self-conscious

2. Which of the following would be the best response by a nursing assistant if a resident refuses to take a bath?
   (A) The NA should offer the resident a prize if he will take the bath.
   (B) The NA should explain to the resident why it is wrong not to bathe.
   (C) The NA should respect the resident's wishes, but report the refusal to the nurse.
   (D) The NA should explain that she might lose her job if the resident does not take the bath.

3. A nursing assistant's husband asks her to tell him some personal details about one of her residents. The best response by the NA would be to
   (A) Explain that she cannot talk about the resident
   (B) Tell him a story if he promises to keep it confidential
   (C) Make up a story to tell, so as not to share anything private
   (D) Tell him something that the NA knows that the resident would not mind her sharing

4. If a nursing assistant suspects a resident is being abused, she should
   (A) Open the resident's mail and look through his belongings to find any clues
   (B) Keep watching the resident to make sure her suspicions are correct
   (C) Report it to the nurse immediately
   (D) Check with other nursing assistants to get some advice

6. Describe what happens when a complaint of abuse is made against a nursing assistant

Short Answer

1. What normally happens immediately when a report of abuse against a nursing assistant is made?

_____

_____

_____

_____

_____

_____

7. Explain how disputes may be resolved and identify the ombudsman's role

Multiple Choice

1. One task of an ombudsman is to
   (A) Decide which special diet is right for a resident
   (B) Investigate and resolve resident complaints
   (C) Diagnose disease and prescribe medication
   (D) Check a resident's vital signs and report to the nurse

2. An ombudsman is assigned by law as the _____ advocate for residents.
   (A) Litigious
   (B) Liable
   (C) Lawyer
   (D) Legal

3. Ombudsmen are in facilities to assist and support
   (A) Administrators
   (B) Directors of nursing
   (C) Residents
   (D) Nursing assistants

Name: _____

8. Explain HIPAA and list ways to protect residents' privacy

Multiple Choice

1. What is the purpose of the Health Insurance Portability and Accountability Act (HIPAA)?
   (A) To monitor quality of care in facilities
   (B) To protect and secure the privacy of health information
   (C) To reduce incidents of abuse in facilities
   (D) To provide health insurance for uninsured elderly people

2. What is included under protected health information (PHI)?
   (A) Patient's favorite food
   (B) Patient's favorite color
   (C) Patient's social security number
   (D) Patient's library card number

3. What is the correct response by a nursing assistant if someone who is not directly involved with a resident's care asks for a resident's PHI?
   (A) Give them the information
   (B) Ask the resident if they may have the information
   (C) Ask them to send a written request for the information
   (D) Tell them that the information is confidential and cannot be given out

4. Which of the following is one way to keep private health information confidential?
   (A) Making comments about residents on Twitter
   (B) Discussing residents' progress with a coworker in a restaurant
   (C) Using confidential rooms for reporting on residents
   (D) Only discussing residents' conditions with trusted family members

5. The abbreviation for a law that was enacted as a part of the American Recovery and Reinvestment Act of 2009 to expand the protection and security of consumers' electronic health records (EHR) is called
   (A) HISEAL
   (B) HITECH
   (C) HIHELP
   (D) HIQUIET

9. Explain the Patient Self-Determination Act (PSDA) and discuss advance directives and related medical orders

Matching
Use each letter only once.

1. _____ Advance directives

2. _____ Durable power of attorney for health care

3. _____ Do-not-resuscitate (DNR) order

4. _____ Living will

5. _____ Physician Orders for Life-Sustaining Treatment (POLST)

(A) A signed, dated, and witnessed legal document that appoints someone else to make medical decisions for a person in the event he or she becomes unable to do so

(B) Outlines the medical care that a person wants, or does not want, in case he or she becomes unable to make those decisions; may also be called medical directive or directive to physicians

(C) Legal documents that allow people to choose what medical care they wish to have if they cannot make those decisions themselves

(D) A medical order that specifies treatments a person wants when he or she is very ill; decisions are based on conversations with health-care providers

(E) A medical order that instructs medical professionals not to perform CPR (cardio-pulmonary resuscitation) if breathing or the heartbeat stops

4

Communication and Cultural Diversity

1. Define *communication*

Short Answer

1. List the three basic steps of communication.

    _____

    _____

    _____

    _____

    _____

2. Why is feedback an important part of communication?

    _____

    _____

    _____

    _____

    _____

    _____

3. With whom must nursing assistants be able to communicate?

    _____

    _____

    _____

    _____

    _____

    _____

    _____

Multiple Choice

4. Which three things are needed for communication to take place?
    (A) Signs, symbols, and drawings
    (B) Sender, receiver, and feedback
    (C) Supervisor, residents, and family members
    (D) Loud voice, ability to speak, resident's chart

5. The three-step process of communication occurs
    (A) Only once
    (B) Over and over
    (C) Only in formal meetings with the care team
    (D) In a different order every time

2. Explain verbal and nonverbal communication

Multiple Choice

1. Which of the following is an example of nonverbal communication?
    (A) Asking for a glass of water
    (B) Pointing to a glass of water
    (C) Screaming for a glass of water
    (D) Saying, "I do not like water."

2. Verbal communication includes
    (A) Facial expressions
    (B) Nodding one's head
    (C) Speaking
    (D) Shrugging one's shoulders

3. Types of nonverbal communication include
    (A) Speaking
    (B) Facial expressions
    (C) Yelling
    (D) Oral reports

Name: _____

4. Which of the following is an example of a confusing or conflicting message (saying one thing and meaning another)?
   (A) Mr. Carter smiles happily and tells his nursing assistant he is excited because his daughter is coming to visit.
   (B) Mrs. Sanchez looks like she is in pain. When her nursing assistant asks her about it, Mrs. Sanchez tells her that her back has been bothering her.
   (C) Ms. Jones agrees with her nursing assistant when she says it is a nice day, but Ms. Jones looks angry.
   (D) Mr. Lee will not watch his favorite TV show. He says he is a little depressed.

5. In the previous question, how could the nursing assistant clarify the confusing or conflicting message?
   (A) Tell the person that the NA knows he or she is not telling the truth
   (B) Ignore the conflicting message and accept what the person has said
   (C) Ask the person to repeat what he or she has just said
   (D) State what the NA has observed and ask if the observation is correct

Short Answer
State whether each behavior below sends a positive message or a negative message to the receiver. Write "P" for positive and "N" for negative.

6. _____ Using an impatient tone

7. _____ Smiling

8. _____ Leaning forward in a chair

9. _____ Glancing repeatedly at a watch

10. _____ Sitting up straight

11. _____ Slouching

12. _____ Crossing arms in front of the body

13. _____ Listening carefully

14. _____ Hugging

15. _____ Rolling eyes

3. Describe ways different cultures communicate

Matching
Use each letter only once.

1. _____ Bias

2. _____ Cultural diversity

3. _____ Culture

(A) Different groups of people with varied backgrounds living together in the world

(B) Learned behaviors that are practiced by a group of people and are passed on

(C) Prejudice

Short Answer

4. What are four ways that people communicate nonverbally that are shaped by culture?

_____

_____

_____

_____

_____

5. What are some things that nursing assistants can do to improve awareness of their residents' cultures and needs?

_____

_____

_____

_____

6. Why is it especially important in the United States to be accepting of cultural diversity?

_____

_____

_____

_____

4. Identify barriers to communication

Crossword

Across

3. Type of terminology that may not be understood by residents or their families; NAs should speak in simple, everyday words

5. Types of questions that should be asked because they elicit more than a "yes" or "no" answer

7. Phrases used over and over again that do not really mean anything

Down

1. This type of language, along with gestures and facial expressions, is part of nonverbal communication; NAs should be aware of this when speaking

2. Being this way and taking time to listen when residents are difficult to understand helps promote better communication

4. NAs cannot offer opinions or give this because it is not within their scope of practice

6. Asking this should be avoided when residents make statements because it often makes people feel defensive

8. Along with profanity, these type of words and expressions should not be used by NAs

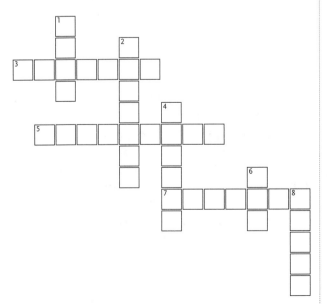

5. List ways to make communication accurate and explain how to develop effective interpersonal relationships

Multiple Choice

1. One way for a nursing assistant to be a good listener is to
   (A) Finish a resident's sentences for him to show that the NA understands what the resident is saying
   (B) Pretend that the NA understands what a resident is saying even if she does not
   (C) Restate the message in the NA's own words
   (D) Fill in any pauses to avoid awkwardness

2. Active listening involves
   (A) Focusing on the sender and giving feedback
   (B) Avoiding speaking to the resident if the NA cannot understand him
   (C) Deciding what the resident is going to say before he says it
   (D) Talking about the NA's personal problems

3. Mrs. Velasco is a new resident who recently moved to the United States. Simon, a nursing assistant, is helping bathe her before bedtime. He notices that she seems to have difficulty speaking English and seems nervous. What can Simon do to make her more comfortable?
   (A) Give her advice about how to fit in better with American culture
   (B) Talk constantly so that she will not have to speak
   (C) Use some words and phrases that he is familiar with in her language
   (D) Avoid speaking to her while giving care

4. When residents report symptoms or feelings, the best response by the NA is to
   (A) Interrupt the resident
   (B) Give medical advice
   (C) Avoid speaking
   (D) Ask for more information

5. Which of the following statements reflects a way for a nursing assistant to have positive relationships with residents?
   (A) The NA should fold her arms in front of her while residents are talking.
   (B) The NA should tell residents she knows exactly how they feel, so residents will feel like they have something in common.
   (C) The NA should ignore a resident's request if she knows she cannot fulfill it.
   (D) The NA should be empathetic and try to understand what residents are going through.

6. Mr. Vernon is an elderly resident who has terminal cancer. He is telling Katie, a nursing assistant, that he is very depressed about dying. He feels he has left many things unfinished. Hearing this makes Katie uncomfortable. Which of the following would be the best response by Katie?
   (A) She should try to ignore what he is saying until he changes the subject.
   (B) She should try to interest him in a brighter subject.
   (C) She should listen to him and ask questions when appropriate.
   (D) She should try to relate to him by telling him she knows just how he feels.

7. Which of the following is the best way for a nursing assistant to refer to a resident?
   (A) Manuel
   (B) Dearie
   (C) Mr. Martinez
   (D) Sweetie

6. Explain the difference between facts and opinions

Fact or Opinion

For each statement, decide whether it is an example of a fact or an opinion. Write F *for fact or* O *for opinion in the space provided.*

1. _____ Mr. Ellington sounds angry.

2. _____ It is better for you to take your bath before you eat.

3. _____ Ms. Crainz will get depressed if she stays in her pajamas all day.

4. _____ Ms. Porter did not drink any of her milk at dinner.

5. _____ I think Mr. Holling is lonely.

6. _____ Mr. Larking's pulse was elevated last night after dinner, but it was back to normal this morning.

7. _____ Mr. Perry and his new roommate are not getting along.

8. _____ Mr. Peterson became agitated while preparing for his bath and refused to wash his hair.

9. _____ Mrs. Myers needs assistance to stand up.

10. _____ Mrs. Myers looks like she is in a lot of pain.

11. _____ Mr. Ford drinks more coffee than is good for him.

12. _____ Mr. Ford drinks three cups of coffee every morning.

Scenario

Karen is a nursing assistant at Greenhollow Extended Care Facility. She has just finished assisting Ms. Lynn, a resident with Alzheimer's disease, with her dinner. She is discussing the events of the meal with her supervisor. Read Karen's statement. Indicate which parts of her report are statements of fact and which are statements of opinion.

"Ms. Lynn was grouchy at dinner today. She said that she did not like the peas and that the milk she has been drinking makes her nauseous. Actually, she did look a little queasy. She liked the meatloaf, but she did not like the peas or the milk. She ate all of the meat, but none of the peas. She only had two sips of milk. During dessert, she got a little depressed. She stopped talking to me and the other residents and only had one bite of her brownie."

_____

_____

_____

_____
_____
_____
_____
_____
_____
_____
_____
_____
_____

16. _____ Coughing

17. _____ Fruity breath

18. _____ Itchy arm

Labeling
Looking at the diagram, list examples of observations using each sense.

Smell: _____
_____
_____
_____

Sight: _____
_____
_____

Hearing: _____
_____
_____

Touch: _____
_____
_____
_____

7. Explain objective and subjective information and describe how to observe and report accurately

Short Answer
For each of the following, decide whether it is an objective observation (you can see, hear, smell, or touch it) or a subjective observation (the resident must tell you about it). Write O for objective and S for subjective.

1. _____ Skin rash

2. _____ Crying

3. _____ Rapid pulse

4. _____ Headache

5. _____ Nausea

6. _____ Vomiting

7. _____ Swelling

8. _____ Cloudy urine

9. _____ Wheezing

10. _____ Feeling sad

11. _____ Red area on skin

12. _____ Fever

13. _____ Dizziness

14. _____ Chest pain

15. _____ Toothache

8. Explain how to communicate with other team members

Multiple Choice

1. When giving information about a resident to other members of the care team, a nursing assistant should
   (A) Use a code name to discuss the resident in front of other residents
   (B) Make a possible diagnosis of the resident's condition
   (C) Share information with anyone who asks about the resident's condition
   (D) Make sure that she respects the resident's right to privacy

2. One health professional who is able to give a resident's family and friends information about any new diagnoses is a(n)
   (A) Nurse
   (B) Nursing assistant
   (C) Activities director
   (D) Music therapist

9. Describe basic medical terminology and abbreviations

Matching

For each of the following abbreviations, write the letter of the correct term from the list below. Use each letter only once.

1. _____ ac, AC
2. _____ amb
3. _____ BM
4. _____ C
5. _____ c/o
6. _____ CPR
7. _____ F
8. _____ ft
9. _____ hs, HS
10. _____ inc
11. _____ I&O
12. _____ NPO
13. _____ OOB
14. _____ pc, p.c.
15. _____ prn, PRN
16. _____ PWB
17. _____ ROM
18. _____ SOB
19. _____ vs, VS
20. _____ w/c, W/C

(A) Fahrenheit degree

(B) Hours sleep

(C) After meals

(D) Nothing by mouth

(E) Bowel movement

(F) Cardiopulmonary resuscitation

(G) Complains of

(H) Range of motion

(I) Partial-weight-bearing

(J) Vital signs

(K) Shortness of breath

(L) Before meals

(M) Foot

(N) Wheelchair

(O) As necessary

(P) Intake and output

(Q) Celsius degree

(R) Out of bed

(S) Incontinent

(T) Ambulate, ambulatory

10. Explain how to give and receive an accurate report of a resident's status

Multiple Choice

1. Which of the following is true of oral reports?
    (A) Nursing assistants should use facts when making oral reports.
    (B) Nursing assistants should use opinions when making oral reports.
    (C) Nursing assistants should make oral reports directly to residents' families.
    (D) Nursing assistants do not need to make oral reports; they only need to complete written reports.

2. Which of the following should be reported to the nurse immediately?
    (A) Trouble sleeping
    (B) Falls
    (C) Visits from family
    (D) Requests for help getting to the toilet

3. What is the best way for a nursing assistant to remember important details for an oral report?
    (A) Rely on his memory
    (B) Repeat the information to a friend
    (C) Write notes and use them for his report
    (D) Ask another nursing assistant to remind him

11. Explain documentation and describe related terms and forms

Multiple Choice

1. The large amount of time that a nursing assistant spends with residents will allow her to
   (A) Diagnose illnesses
   (B) Determine treatments
   (C) Notice things about residents that other care team members may not notice
   (D) Give medical advice

2. Which of the following statements is true of a resident's medical chart?
   (A) A medical chart is the legal record of a resident's care.
   (B) Not all care needs to be documented.
   (C) Documentation can be put off until the next day if a nursing assistant is busy.
   (D) Medical charts are not considered legal documents.

3. When should care be documented?
   (A) Before care is given
   (B) Immediately after care is given
   (C) At the end of the day
   (D) Whenever there is time

Short Answer

Convert the following times to military time:

4. 2:10 p.m. _____

5. 4:30 a.m. _____

6. 10:00 a.m. _____

7. 8:25 p.m. _____

Convert the following times to regular time:

8. 0600 _____

9. 2320 _____

10. 1927 _____

11. 1800 _____

12. Describe incident reporting and recording

Multiple Choice

1. An incident is
   (A) An accident or unexpected event in the course of care
   (B) Any interaction between residents and staff
   (C) A normal part of facility routines
   (D) Any event in a resident's day

2. Which of the following would be considered an incident?
   (A) A resident complains of a headache.
   (B) A resident falls but is okay after the fall.
   (C) A resident wants to watch TV in the common living area.
   (D) A resident needs to be transferred from his bed to a chair.

3. Incidents should be reported to
   (A) The resident's family
   (B) The charge nurse
   (C) All staff on duty at the time of the incident
   (D) The doctor on call

True or False

4. _____ Documentation of incidents helps protect the resident, the employer, and individual staff members.

5. _____ The information in an incident report is confidential.

6. _____ If an NA does not actually see an incident but arrives after it has already occurred, she should document what she thinks happened.

7. _____ The documentation of an incident should include who the nursing assistant thinks could be responsible for the incident.

8. _____ Incident reports should be factual.

9. _____ If a resident who is supposed to eat a low-sodium meal eats a regular, unrestricted meal, an incident report does not need to be completed.

10. _____ If an NA receives an injury on the job, he should file an incident report.

Name: _____

13. Demonstrate effective communication on the telephone

Scenarios

Read the following telephone conversations and think about how the nursing assistant could have better presented herself on the phone.

Example #1 Making a call from a facility

Hi, who's this?

Could you get Ms. Crier on the phone, please? I need to talk to her.

She's not there? Do you know where she is? I really have to talk to her right now. My resident asked me to call her to see if she can come visit today. She's really lonely and needs a visitor.

Okay, well tell her Ella called and have her call me back. Ella Ferguson. The number? I don't remember what it is. Just look up Whispering Pines Nursing Facility.

I don't know how much longer I'll be here, but have her call me as soon as possible. Bye.

1. What did the nursing assistant do incorrectly in this phone conversation?

   _____

   _____

   _____

   _____

   _____

   _____

   _____

   _____

   _____

   _____

Example #2 Answering a call at a facility

Hello? Who? Julie Lee? No, she can't come to the phone right now. She's on her break outside and is smoking a cigarette. Who's calling?

And your number?

Can I tell her what this is about?

Okay. I'll give her the message. Goodbye.

2. What did the nursing assistant do incorrectly in this phone conversation?

   _____

   _____

   _____

   _____

   _____

   _____

   _____

   _____

   _____

14. Explain the resident call system

Multiple Choice

1. How do residents signal staff that they need assistance?
   (A) By calling out their names as they see them
   (B) By calling the nurses' station on the phone
   (C) By using a signal light or call light
   (D) By calling family members on the phone

2. When is it acceptable for a nursing assistant to ignore a call light?
   (A) When she has just left a resident's room
   (B) When she is very busy
   (C) When the resident signaling is not assigned to her
   (D) Never

3. Call lights should be placed
   (A) Near the door of the resident's room
   (B) In a common area of the floor
   (C) Within reach of the resident's stronger hand
   (D) In any location that is convenient

15. List guidelines for communicating with residents with special needs

Multiple Choice

Hearing Impairment

1. To best communicate with a resident who has a hearing impairment, the nursing assistant should
   (A) Use short sentences and simple words
   (B) Shout
   (C) Approach the resident from behind
   (D) Raise the pitch of her voice

2. If a resident is difficult to understand, the NA should
   (A) Pretend to understand the resident so as not to hurt his feelings
   (B) Mouth the words in an exaggerated way so that the resident will mimic that behavior next time
   (C) Ask the resident to repeat what he said, and then tell the resident what the NA thinks she heard
   (D) Ask the resident to speak up

3. Hearing aids should be cleaned
   (A) Every couple of hours
   (B) Daily
   (C) Once a week
   (D) When the resident is sleeping

Multiple Choice

Vision Impairment

4. The ability to see objects in the distance better than objects nearby is
   (A) Closesightedness
   (B) Farsightedness
   (C) Nearsightedness
   (D) Neurosightedness

5. Which of the following would the best way for a nursing assistant to orient a resident who is visually impaired to a step in a room?
   (A) Look at the step below you.
   (B) Watch out for the step below.
   (C) There is a step at twelve o'clock.
   (D) Visualize a step in front of you.

6. When entering the room of a resident who is visually impaired, the nursing assistant should
   (A) Touch the resident, then identify herself
   (B) Be quiet so as not to disturb the resident
   (C) Wait until she is very close to the resident, then touch the resident on the arm
   (D) Knock on the door and then identify herself

7. When helping a resident who is visually impaired walk, the nursing assistant should
   (A) Walk slightly in front of the resident
   (B) Walk slightly behind the resident
   (C) Walk on the resident's stronger side
   (D) Gently push the resident forward

Matching

Cerebrovascular Accident (CVA) or Stroke
Use each letter only once.

8. _____ Cerebrovascular accident (CVA)

9. _____ Dysphagia

10. _____ Emotional lability

11. _____ Expressive aphasia

12. _____ Hemiparesis

13. _____ Hemiplegia

14. _____ Receptive aphasia

(A) Occurs when blood supply is blocked or a blood vessel leaks or ruptures within the brain

(B) Weakness on one side of the body

(C) Paralysis on one side of the body

(D) Trouble communicating thoughts through speech or writing

(E) Difficulty understanding spoken or written words

(F) Inappropriate or unprovoked emotional responses

(G) Difficulty swallowing

Fill in the Blank

15. Keep questions and directions

    _____.

16. Ask questions that can be answered with a

    _____ or

    _____ .

17. Refer to the side of the resident's body with weakness or paralysis as the

    _____ or

    _____ side.

18. Keep the _____ within reach of resident.

19. Use gestures, pointing, and

    _____

    boards to aid communication.

20. Both verbal and _____ communication can express a positive attitude.

True or False

Combativeness and/or Anger

21. _____ Combative behavior can be verbal as well as physical.

22. _____ Combative behavior is usually a reaction to the specific caregiver that is with the resident at a particular time.

23. _____ As long as the nursing assistant is not upset by it, combative behavior does not need to be reported.

24. _____ It is acceptable to hit a resident if the resident hits the nursing assistant first.

25. _____ Presenting logical arguments is a good way to counter combative behavior.

26. _____ Anger may be expressed through violent, aggressive behavior or by withdrawal or sulking.

27. _____ Using silence may allow a resident to express why she is angry.

28. _____ Assertive behavior includes expressing thoughts, feelings, and beliefs in a direct and honest way.

True or False

Inappropriate Behavior

29. _____ Inappropriate behavior includes comments as well as physical actions.

30. _____ Illness, dementia, or medication may cause inappropriate behavior.

31. _____ Overreacting to inappropriate behavior may actually reinforce the behavior.

32. _____ As long as a resident's behavior is harmless, the nursing assistant does not need to report it.

5

Infection Prevention and Control

1. Define *infection prevention* and discuss types of infections

Matching
Use each letter only once.

1. _____ Healthcare-associated infection

2. _____ Infection

3. _____ Infection prevention

4. _____ Localized infection

5. _____ Microorganism/microbe

6. _____ Pathogen

7. _____ Systemic infection

(A) Methods practiced in healthcare facilities to prevent and control the spread of disease

(B) A harmful microorganism

(C) Infections acquired in healthcare settings during the delivery of medical care

(D) A living thing that is only visible under a microscope

(E) An infection that is in the bloodstream and is spread throughout the body

(F) Occurs when pathogens invade the body and multiply

(G) An infection that is limited to a specific location in the body

2. Describe the chain of infection

Multiple Choice

1. The following are necessary links in the chain of infection. Which link is broken by wearing gloves, thus preventing the spread of disease?
    (A) Reservoir (place where the pathogen lives and grows)
    (B) Mode of transmission (a way for the disease to spread)
    (C) Susceptible host (person who is likely to get the disease)
    (D) Portal of exit (body opening that allows pathogens to leave)

2. The following are necessary links in the chain of infection. By getting a vaccination shot for hepatitis B, which link will a person affect to prevent him from getting this disease?
    (A) Reservoir (place where the pathogen lives and grows)
    (B) Mode of transmission (a way for the disease to spread)
    (C) Susceptible host (person who is likely to get the disease)
    (D) Portal of exit (body opening that allows pathogens to leave)

3. Which of the following is the primary route of disease transmission within the healthcare setting?
    (A) The hands of healthcare workers
    (B) The carts that contain residents' meals
    (C) The utility rooms where linen is stored
    (D) The nurses' station where the charts are kept

4. In what type of environment do microorganisms grow best?
   (A) In a warm, moist place
   (B) In a bright place
   (C) In a cool, dry place
   (D) In a frozen place

3. Explain why the elderly are at a higher risk for infection

True or False

1. ____ The elderly have a higher risk for infection than younger people.

2. ____ It is normal for a person's immune system to grow weaker as he or she ages.

3. ____ Blood circulation increases as a person ages.

4. ____ Limited mobility increases the risk of pressure injuries among the elderly.

5. ____ Nutrition is not normally a factor in preventing infections.

6. ____ The elderly are less likely than younger people to have healthcare-associated infections.

7. ____ Infections are less dangerous in the elderly than they are in younger people.

8. ____ Nursing assistants play an important role in protecting elderly residents from infections.

4. Explain Standard Precautions

True or False

1. ____ Following Standard Precautions means treating all blood, body fluids, non-intact skin, and mucous membranes as if they were infected.

2. ____ Under Standard Precautions, body fluids do not include saliva.

3. ____ A nursing assistant can usually tell if someone is infectious just by looking at him.

4. ____ A nursing assistant should wash her hands before donning (putting on) gloves.

5. ____ A nursing assistant should carefully recap used syringes before putting them in a biohazard container.

6. ____ Giving mouth care is one task that requires a nursing assistant to wear gloves.

7. ____ A mask and protective goggles may need to be worn when emptying a bedpan.

8. ____ Waste that contains blood can be disposed of in the regular trash can.

Multiple Choice

9. Standard Precautions should be practiced
   (A) Only on people who look like they have a bloodborne disease
   (B) On every single person under a nursing assistant's care
   (C) Only on people who request that the nursing assistant follow them
   (D) Only on people who have tuberculosis

10. Standard Precautions include the following measures:
    (A) Washing hands after taking off gloves but not before putting on gloves
    (B) Wearing gloves if there is a possibility of coming into contact with blood, body fluids, mucous membranes, or broken skin
    (C) Touching body fluids with bare hands
    (D) Disposing of sharps in plastic bags

11. Which of the following is true of Transmission-Based Precautions?
    (A) A nursing assistant does not need to practice Standard Precautions if he practices Transmission-Based Precautions.
    (B) They are exactly the same as Standard Precautions.
    (C) They are practiced in addition to Standard Precautions.
    (D) They are never practiced at the same time that Standard Precautions are used.

12. How should sharps such as needles be discarded?
    (A) Sharps should be placed in blue recycling containers.
    (B) Sharps should be placed in break room trash containers.
    (C) Sharps should be placed inside used gloves and then put in the trash receptacle.
    (D) Sharps should be placed in biohazard containers.

13. The Occupational Safety and Health Administration (OSHA) is a federal government agency that protects workers from
    (A) Unfair employment practices
    (B) Sexual harassment
    (C) Workplace violence
    (D) Hazards on the job

5. Explain hand hygiene and identify when to wash hands

Multiple Choice

1. A nursing assistant (NA) will come into contact with microorganisms
   (A) Only in public areas of the facility
   (B) Only during direct contact with residents
   (C) Only during personal care procedures
   (D) Every time the NA touches something

2. Centers for Disease Control and Prevention (CDC) defines hand hygiene as
   (A) Handwashing with soap and water and using alcohol-based hand rubs
   (B) Using only alcohol-based hand rubs when hands are visibly soiled
   (C) Rinsing hands with cold water
   (D) Not washing hands more than once per day

3. Alcohol-based hand rubs are used
   (A) With water for maximum effectiveness
   (B) When facilities have run out of antimicrobial soap
   (C) To prevent dry, cracked skin
   (D) In addition to washing with soap and water

4. Why should a nursing assistant not wear artificial nails to work?
   (A) Residents may not like them.
   (B) They may be damaged during resident care.
   (C) They harbor bacteria and increase risk of contamination.
   (D) They may be torn or damaged by frequent handwashing.

5. How long should a nursing assistant use friction when lathering and washing her hands?
   (A) 2 minutes
   (B) 5 seconds
   (C) 18 seconds
   (D) 20 seconds

6. Discuss the use of personal protective equipment (PPE) in facilities

Short Answer
Make a check mark (✓) next to the tasks that require a nursing assistant to wear gloves.

1. _____ Contact with body fluids

2. _____ When the NA may touch blood

3. _____ Brushing a resident's hair

4. _____ Answering the telephone

5. _____ Assisting with perineal care

6. _____ Washing vegetables

7. _____ Giving a massage to a resident who has acne on her back

8. _____ Assisting with mouth care

9. _____ Shaving a resident

Multiple Choice

10. What type of personal protective equipment may be needed when caring for a resident with a respiratory illness?
    (A) Eyeglasses and mask
    (B) Mask and foot covering
    (C) Eyeglasses and gloves
    (D) Mask and goggles

11. What type of personal protective equipment is used most often by caregivers?
    (A) Gloves
    (B) Mask
    (C) Face shield
    (D) Goggles

12. How many times can a gown be worn before it needs to be discarded?
    (A) One time
    (B) Two times
    (C) Three times
    (D) Four times

13. If blood or body fluids may be splashed or sprayed into the eye area, proper protection for the eyes is
    (A) Gloves
    (B) Mask
    (C) Gown
    (D) Goggles

Short Answer

After Zoe washes her hands, she will put on her personal protective equipment. She is going into an area in which she needs to use Transmission-Based Precautions, so she will wear a gown, a mask, and goggles in addition to her gloves. Read the steps she takes and write down anything she does incorrectly.

14. First Zoe puts on her gown. She holds it out in front of her and shakes it open. She slips her arms into the sleeves and then ties the neck ties in a secure knot so that it will not come untied while she is working. She reaches behind her and, making sure all of her clothing is covered, ties the back ties.

    _____
    _____
    _____
    _____
    _____
    _____
    _____
    _____
    _____
    _____

15. Zoe then puts on her mask. Being careful not to touch the mask where it touches her face, she ties the bottom strings first and then the top strings. She then puts on her goggles, making sure they fit snugly over her eyeglasses.

    _____

_____
_____
_____
_____
_____
_____
_____
_____
_____

16. Zoe is right-handed, so she will put on her right glove first. She then uses her gloved hand to put on her other glove. She holds her hands out in front of her to smooth out the folds in the gloves. She looks closely at the gloves for tears or holes. She sees an area that is discolored, but it is very small, so she decides to wear the glove anyway. She pulls the sleeves of her gown over the cuffs of the gloves and is ready to get to work.

    _____
    _____
    _____
    _____
    _____
    _____
    _____
    _____
    _____
    _____
    _____

Short Answer

17. What is the correct order for donning (putting on) PPE (gloves, mask, gown, goggles)?

1st _____

2nd _____

Name: _____

3rd _____

4th _____

18. What is the correct order for doffing (removing) PPE (gloves, mask, gown, goggles)?

1st _____

2nd _____

3rd _____

4th _____

7. List guidelines for handling equipment and linen

Matching
Use each letter only once.

1. _____ Clean

2. _____ Dirty

3. _____ Disinfection

4. _____ Disposable

5. _____ Sterilization

(A) A measure that destroys all microorganisms, including pathogens

(B) A process that kills pathogens, but does not destroy all pathogens

(C) Only to be used once and then discarded

(D) In health care, objects that have not been contaminated with pathogens

(E) In health care, objects that have been contaminated with pathogens

Multiple Choice

6. How many times can disposable equipment be used before it needs to be discarded?
   (A) Three times
   (B) One time
   (C) Two times if it is washed in between uses
   (D) Indefinitely if it is sterilized in between uses

7. How should dirty linen be rolled or folded?
   (A) Dirty area is inside
   (B) Clean area is inside
   (C) Dirty area is on top
   (D) Clean area is tucked underneath dirty area

8. Dirty linen should be
   (A) Shaken to remove contaminants before taking it to the soiled linen room
   (B) Carried away from the NA's uniform
   (C) Bagged outside of the resident's room
   (D) Stored in the same area as clean linen

8. Explain how to handle spills

True or False

1. _____ A nursing assistant does not need to wear gloves to clean up a very small spill.

2. _____ Disinfectant should be placed directly on the spilled fluid before absorbing and removing the fluid.

3. _____ A nursing assistant should use her hands to pick up large pieces of broken glass and use a broom and dustpan for smaller pieces.

4. _____ Waste containing blood or body fluids should be disposed of in the resident's trash can and the housekeeping department should be notified.

5. _____ An absorbing powder may be used to absorb the spill before removing it.

9. Explain Transmission-Based Precautions

Short Answer
List the type of precaution being described in each phrase below. Use an A for Airborne Precautions, a C for Contact Precautions, and a D for Droplet Precautions. Each letter may be used more than once.

1. _____ Transmission can occur when touching a contaminated area on the resident's body

2. ____ Used when there is a risk of spreading an infection by direct contact with a person or object

3. ____ Used to guard against tuberculosis

4. ____ Covering the nose and mouth with a tissue when a person sneezes or coughs and washing hands immediately after sneezing are parts of these precautions

5. ____ Helps prevent the spread of *Clostridium difficile* (*C. diff*) and conjunctivitis

6. ____ Used when the microorganisms are spread by droplets in the air that travel only short distances (normally not more than six feet)

7. ____ Microorganisms can be spread by coughing, sneezing, talking, laughing, or suctioning

8. ____ Helps prevent the spread of illnesses transmitted through the air

9. ____ Helps protects against transmission of influenza

10. ____ May require the use of a special mask, such as an N95 or HEPA mask

Multiple Choice

11. Transmission-Based Precautions are used
   (A) With every resident under a nursing assistant's care
   (B) In addition to Standard Precautions
   (C) Instead of Standard Precautions
   (D) When a nursing assistant decides that they are appropriate for particular residents

12. Dedicated equipment refers to
   (A) Equipment that is used by multiple residents
   (B) Equipment donated to one resident by another resident and/or his family
   (C) Equipment that is disposable
   (D) Equipment that is used by only one resident

13. Which of the following is true of wearing personal protective equipment (PPE) while caring for residents in isolation?
   (A) Nursing assistants will have to decide for themselves which PPE they must wear while caring for residents in isolation.
   (B) Nursing assistants should remove PPE before exiting a resident's room.
   (C) Nursing assistants will always wear the same PPE while caring for all residents in isolation.
   (D) Nursing assistants should remove PPE after exiting a resident's room.

14. When a resident is in isolation,
   (A) She should be avoided until the time in isolation is completed.
   (B) Nursing assistants will be unable to perform care for her.
   (C) She needs to feel that her feelings are understood by care team members.
   (D) Nursing assistants should not practice Standard Precautions.

10. Define *bloodborne pathogens* and describe two major bloodborne diseases

Multiple Choice

1. Bloodborne diseases can be transmitted by
   (A) Infected blood entering the bloodstream
   (B) Hugging a person with a bloodborne disease
   (C) Being in the same room as a person with a bloodborne disease
   (D) Talking to a person with a bloodborne disease

2. In health care, the most common way to be infected by a bloodborne disease is by
   (A) Contact with infected blood or certain body fluids
   (B) Sharing contaminated needles between residents
   (C) Being in the same room as a resident with a bloodborne disease
   (D) Sexual contact with an infected resident

3. How does the human immunodeficiency virus (HIV) affect the body?
   (A) It cuts off blood supply to the brain.
   (B) It causes inadequate nutritional intake by damaging the gastrointestinal system.
   (C) It causes diabetes in otherwise healthy people.
   (D) It weakens the immune system so that the body cannot fight infection.

4. Which of the following is true of hepatitis B (HBV)?
   (A) HBV is caused by fecal-oral contamination.
   (B) There is no vaccine for HBV.
   (C) HBV is caused by jaundice.
   (D) HBV can be transmitted through blood or needles that are contaminated with the virus.

5. Employers must offer a free vaccine to protect nursing assistants from
   (A) AIDS
   (B) Hepatitis B
   (C) Hepatitis C
   (D) All bloodborne diseases

11. Explain OSHA's Bloodborne Pathogens Standard

Multiple Choice

1. The Bloodborne Pathogens Standard is a law that requires that
   (A) Healthcare employers must have a written exposure control plan designed to eliminate or reduce employee exposure to infectious material
   (B) Healthcare employers must only accept residents who are healthy upon admission
   (C) Healthcare employers must charge employees a discounted fee for hepatitis B vaccinations
   (D) Healthcare employers must disclose information about residents' bloodborne diseases to the public

2. Which of the following does OSHA consider a significant exposure?
   (A) NA is stuck by a needle
   (B) Resident makes a complaint against an NA
   (C) NA does not discard her personal protective equipment properly
   (D) NA was recently diagnosed with cancer

3. According to OSHA, employers must give all employees, residents, and visitors _____ to use when needed.
   (A) Syringe caps
   (B) Manual Data Set (MDS) assessments
   (C) Personal protective equipment (PPE)
   (D) Medical charts

4. Why is it important for an employee to report any potential exposures immediately?
   (A) So that the employee can be terminated to avoid infecting others
   (B) To avoid any appearance of negligence on the part of the facility
   (C) To protect the employee's health and the health of others
   (D) So that the employee can warn residents of a possible epidemic

12. Define *tuberculosis* and list infection prevention guidelines

Multiple Choice

1. Tuberculosis may be transmitted
   (A) By coughing
   (B) By dancing
   (C) By wearing gloves
   (D) Through a protective mask

2. Tuberculosis is
   (A) A bloodborne disease
   (B) An airborne disease
   (C) A non-infectious disease
   (D) An untreatable disease

3. Someone with latent TB infection
   (A) Shows symptoms
   (B) Infects others within three feet
   (C) Cannot infect others
   (D) Infects others who have a compromised immune system

4. A person with TB disease
   (A) Can infect others
   (B) Does not show symptoms
   (C) Must eat a pureed diet
   (D) Cannot infect others

5. TB disease is more likely to develop in people
   (A) Who live near the mountains
   (B) Whose relatives had it when they were kids
   (C) Who have weakened immune systems
   (D) Who work alone

6. The word *resistant* in multidrug-resistant TB (MDR-TB) means that
   (A) Medications can no longer kill the specific bacteria
   (B) The infected person does not want to treat his or her disease
   (C) Doctors do not know what causes the disease
   (D) The infected person will die from the disease

13. Discuss MRSA, VRE, and C. *Difficile*

True or False

1. _____ Methicillin-resistant *Staphylococcus aureus* (MRSA) is almost always spread by direct physical contact.

2. _____ Once vancomycin-resistant *enterococcus* (VRE) is established, it is relatively easy to get rid of it.

3. _____ MRSA can be spread through indirect contact by touching objects contaminated by a person with MRSA.

4. _____ Handwashing will not help control the spread of MRSA.

5. _____ VRE causes life-threatening infections in people with weak immune systems.

6. _____ Frequent handwashing can help prevent the spread of VRE.

7. _____ Handwashing and proper handling of contaminated wastes can help prevent *Clostridium difficile* (C. *difficile*).

8. _____ Increasing the use of antibiotics helps lower the risk of developing C. *difficile* diarrhea.

9. _____ Both hand sanitizers and washing hands with soap and water are considered equally effective when dealing with C. *difficile*.

14. List employer and employee responsibilities for infection prevention

Short Answer
Read the following and mark ER for employer or EE for employee to show who is responsible for infection prevention.

1. _____ Immediately report any exposure to infection, blood, or body fluids.

2. _____ Provide personal protective equipment for use and train how to properly use it.

3. _____ Follow all facility policies and procedures.

4. _____ Take advantage of the free hepatitis B vaccination.

5. _____ Provide continuing in-service education about infection prevention.

6. _____ Establish infection prevention procedures and an exposure control plan.

7. _____ Follow resident care plans and assignments.

8. _____ Participate in continuing in-service education programs covering infection prevention.

9. _____ Use provided personal protective equipment as indicated or as appropriate.

10. _____ Provide free hepatitis B vaccinations.

6

Safety and Body Mechanics

1. Identify the persons at greatest risk for accidents and describe accident prevention guidelines

Short Answer

1. Why do the elderly have more safety concerns than younger people?

_____

_____

_____

_____

_____

_____

2. What is the key to safety in facilities?

_____

_____

_____

_____

Multiple Choice

Falls

3. Generally speaking, in what position should a bed be left after a nursing assistant has finished giving care?
   (A) Upright position
   (B) Lowest position
   (C) About two inches away from the wall
   (D) Highest position

4. If a resident starts to fall after standing up, the nursing assistant should
   (A) Use her body to slide the resident to the floor
   (B) Push the resident gently into her wheelchair
   (C) Have the resident use the nearest piece of heavy furniture to brace herself
   (D) Prop the resident up to try to stop the fall

5. Which of the following should always be locked before giving care?
   (A) Bathroom door
   (B) Bedside table
   (C) Bed wheels
   (D) Door to the resident's room

Multiple Choice

Burns/Scalds

6. Those at greatest risk for burns are
   (A) Middle-aged adults who are not active
   (B) Young adults
   (C) People who have a loss of sensation
   (D) Teenagers who are careless

7. Scalds are burns caused by
   (A) Hot liquids
   (B) Lye
   (C) Hot irons
   (D) Heating devices

8. How long does it take for a serious burn to occur with a liquid at a temperature of 140°F?
   (A) 5 seconds or less
   (B) 10 seconds or less
   (C) 30 seconds or less
   (D) 60 seconds or less

Name: _____

9. How should the nursing assistant check the temperature of hot water?
   (A) Put her hand in the water
   (B) Estimate the temperature based on how long it has been heating
   (C) Use a water thermometer
   (D) Use a stethoscope

10. What should a nursing assistant do if an appliance has a frayed cord or looks unsafe?
    (A) The NA should report it immediately and remove it from the area.
    (B) The NA should report it immediately but continue to use it until it is replaced.
    (C) The NA should try to repair it himself if he is handy.
    (D) The NA should continue to use it; it has probably already been reported.

11. When serving hot liquids to residents, the nursing assistant should
    (A) Pour hot drinks as close as possible to residents
    (B) Pour hot drinks away from residents
    (C) Keep hot liquids close to the edges of tables
    (D) Ask residents to stand up before serving hot drinks

Short Answer

Resident Identification

12. What can happen if a nursing assistant does not identify a resident before mealtimes or giving care?

_____

_____

_____

_____

13. How should a nursing assistant identify a resident before placing a meal tray?

_____

_____

_____

_____

_____

True or False

Choking

14. _____ Choking can occur while swallowing medication.

15. _____ People who are weak may choke on their own saliva.

16. _____ To avoid choking, residents should eat in a semi-reclined position.

17. _____ Liquids thickened to the consistency of honey are easier to swallow.

Short Answer

Poisoning

18. List five items in a facility that can cause poisoning.

_____

_____

_____

_____

_____

_____

_____

_____

_____

_____

True or False

Cuts/Scrapes

19. _____ Cuts most often occur in a person's bedroom.

20. _____ Scissors should be put away immediately after use.

21. _____ The correct way to move a wheelchair is for a nursing assistant to push it forward, rather than pulling it.

22. _____ Residents in wheelchairs should be facing the back of the elevator when riding in elevators.

2. List safety guidelines for oxygen use

True or False

1. _____ Oxygen therapy is prescribed by a doctor.

2. _____ Nursing assistants are usually responsible for adjusting oxygen settings for residents.

3. _____ Oxygen supports combustion; this means it makes other things burn.

4. _____ A flammable liquid like alcohol is fine to have in a room when oxygen is in use, as long as it is covered.

5. _____ Smoking is allowed near where oxygen is stored as long as the oxygen is not in use.

6. _____ Oxygen should be turned off in the event of a fire.

7. _____ Nursing assistants should check the skin around oxygen masks and tubing for irritation.

8. _____ If a resident has skin irritation around a nasal cannula, the NA should use Vaseline to soften the skin.

3. Explain the Safety Data Sheet (SDS)

Multiple Choice

1. Which of the following is included on a Safety Data Sheet (SDS)?
   (A) Chemical ingredients and dangers
   (B) Correct response to resident abuse
   (C) Fire evacuation procedures
   (D) Safe handling information for restraints

2. Employers must
   (A) Keep SDS information confidential from employees
   (B) Terminate employees who do not know how to use an SDS
   (C) Have an SDS for every chemical used
   (D) Edit an SDS if they do not agree with what is listed

4. Define the term *restraint* and give reasons why restraints were used

Multiple Choice

1. The purpose of restraints is to
   (A) Discipline residents
   (B) Make the nursing assistant's job easier
   (C) Restrict voluntary movement or behavior
   (D) Allow ill residents to be left alone for longer periods of time

2. An example of a physical restraint is
   (A) A bed
   (B) A wheelchair
   (C) Medication
   (D) Raised side rails on a bed

3. A chemical restraint is
   (A) Medication used to control behavior
   (B) Medication used to treat illness
   (C) A medical procedure
   (D) A restraint placed on the person's hands

4. What is one reason the use of restraints has been restricted?
   (A) They were found to be too expensive.
   (B) They were abused by caregivers.
   (C) They were difficult for caregivers to use.
   (D) They were not keeping residents occupied for a long enough period of time.

5. A restraint can be used
   (A) For discipline
   (B) When a doctor has ordered its use
   (C) To stop residents from using call lights
   (D) Whenever staff members are busy

5. List physical and psychological problems associated with restraints

Fill in the Blank
Fill in the blank with some of the problems associated with restraint use.

1. Reduced blood _____

2. Stress on the
   _____

3. Muscle
   _____

4. _____
    injuries

5. Risk of _____

6. Poor _____

7. _____
    disorders

8. Loss of _____
    and loss of

    _____

9. Severe

    _____

6. Discuss restraint alternatives

Multiple Choice

1. Restraint-free care means that
    (A) Restraints are used when nurses request
        they be used
    (B) Restraints are used when necessary for
        safety
    (C) Restraints are never used for any reason
    (D) Restraints are used with permission
        from the resident's family

2. Restraint alternatives are
    (A) Measures used in place of a restraint
    (B) Restraints that keep residents in their
        beds
    (C) Medications used to control a person's
        behavior
    (D) Periods of confining residents to their
        rooms

Short Answer

3. List five alternative actions that help reduce
    the need for a restraint.

    _____

    _____

    _____

    _____

    _____

    _____

_____

_____

7. Describe guidelines for what must be done if a restraint is ordered

Crossword

Across

3. Position in which the hand should be placed
    between the resident and the restraint to
    ensure that the device fits properly and is
    comfortable

4. One color that may indicate skin irritation
    caused by a restraint

5. Before a restraint is applied, the nursing as-
    sistant must make sure there is one of these

Down

1. The minimum number of minutes at which
    a resident in a physical restraint must be
    checked

2. Device that must be placed within a resi-
    dent's reach when the resident is restrained

8. Explain the principles of body mechanics

Labeling
Complete the illustration by labeling each part with the words listed below.

Alignment

Base of support

Center of gravity

Fulcrum

Lever

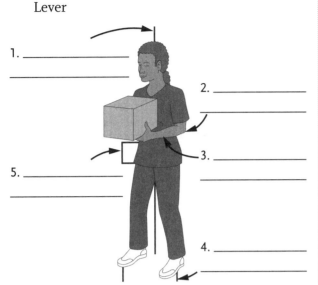

1. _____
_____

2. _____
_____

3. _____
_____

5. _____
_____

4. _____
_____

True or False

6. _____ Nursing assistants are at risk for back injuries and strain.

7. _____ Using proper body mechanics can help save energy and prevent injury.

8. _____ When lifting an object, it is safer to hold it far away from the body.

9. _____ Feet should be pointed toward the object that a person is lifting.

10. _____ Keeping the feet close together gives the body the best base of support and keeps a person more stable.

11. _____ A high center of gravity gives a more stable base of support.

12. _____ Knees should be bent when lifting an object.

9. Apply principles of body mechanics to daily activities

Scenario

Sharon is lifting a large box of supplies from the floor to place on a cart. Keeping her feet together, Sharon bends her knees and uses the muscles in her thighs, upper arms, and shoulders to lift the box. She holds the box at arm's length to place it on the cart. She is careful to move the box and her body at the same time while lifting.

1. What did Sharon do correctly? What should she have done differently?

_____

_____

_____

_____

_____

_____

_____

_____

_____

_____

Fill in the Blank

2. Nursing assistants should avoid _____ at the waist when moving an object; their feet should always _____ toward what they are lifting or moving.

3. When lifting a heavy object from the floor, feet should be spread _____ apart. Knees should be _____.

4. If a resident falls, the nursing assistant should not try to catch her; instead she should help the resident to the _____.

5. Bending from the _____ should be avoided.

6. A bed should be adjusted to a safe working level, which is usually _____ high.

7. A nursing assistant should _____ or slide objects rather than lift them.

8. A nursing assistant should get _____ when possible for lifting or helping residents.

9. When moving a resident, the nursing assistant and the resident should agree on a _____, such as counting to three so that everyone moves together.

10. Identify major causes of fire and list fire safety guidelines

Multiple Choice

1. What is needed for a fire to occur?
   (A) Heat
   (B) Water
   (C) Ice
   (D) Dirt

2. Which of the following is appropriate for a nursing assistant to do if a fire occurs?
   (A) Check for heat coming from a door before opening it
   (B) Take the nearest elevator to the ground floor
   (C) Start running if her clothing is on fire
   (D) Get to the highest point possible in a room

3. Which of the following is considered a potential fire hazard in a facility?
   (A) Oxygen use
   (B) Call light
   (C) Uneaten food
   (D) Specimen container

Short Answer

4. PASS is an acronym that stands for

   P: _____

   A: _____

   S: _____

   S: _____

5. RACE is an acronym that stands for

   R: _____

   A: _____

   C: _____

   E: _____

6. Explain the fire safety technique *stop, drop, and roll.*

   _____

   _____

   _____

7

Emergency Care and Disaster Preparation

1. Demonstrate how to recognize and respond to medical emergencies

Crossword

Across

4. Being mentally alert and having awareness of surroundings, sensations, and thoughts

6. What a nursing assistant must do after the emergency is over

Down

1. One type of wound that is considered a medical emergency

2. The person who responds to a medical emergency needs to assess the situation and assess this

3. In addition to checking for danger, noticing this is part of assessing the situation during a medical emergency

5. What needs to be reported when documenting an emergency

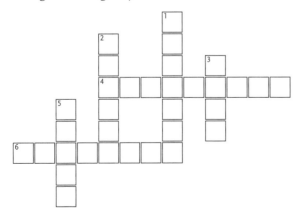

2. Demonstrate knowledge of first aid procedures

Multiple Choice

1. First aid refers to
   - (A) Care given by the first people to respond to an emergency
   - (B) The person with the highest level of medical training who responds to the emergency
   - (C) Any person the victim has given permission to treat him or her during an emergency
   - (D) The first person to give consent to medical professionals for treating the victim

2. If an emergency occurs, the nursing assistant should immediately notify
   - (A) The resident's family
   - (B) The nurse
   - (C) The resident's friends in the facility
   - (D) The resident's clergyperson

3. How can someone usually tell if a person is choking?
   - (A) The choking victim will tell the person.
   - (B) The choking victim will ask for food.
   - (C) The choking victim will put his hands to his throat.
   - (D) The choking victim will throw up.

4. Where should the hands be placed to give abdominal thrusts?
   - (A) Under the person's arms and around his waist
   - (B) Under the person's arms and around his chest
   - (C) Over his shoulders and around his neck
   - (D) Under the person's arms and around his pelvis

5. How does a rescuer obtain consent to give a choking victim abdominal thrusts?
    (A) Rescuer asks victim's spouse to sign a consent form
    (B) Rescuer asks facility administrator, "May I treat this resident who lives at your facility?"
    (C) Rescuer asks his supervisor
    (D) Rescuer asks victim, "Are you choking?"

6. Signs of shock include
    (A) Pale or bluish skin
    (B) Lack of thirst
    (C) Being asleep
    (D) Relaxation

7. If a nursing assistant suspects that a resident is having a heart attack, she should
    (A) Give the resident something cold to drink
    (B) Loosen the clothing around the resident's neck
    (C) Encourage the resident to walk around
    (D) Leave the resident alone to rest

8. To control bleeding, a nursing assistant should
    (A) Use her bare hands to stop it
    (B) Lower the wound below the level of the heart
    (C) Hold a thick pad or clean cloth against the wound and press down hard
    (D) Give the resident an aspirin, which will stop the bleeding

9. Which kind of burn involves just the outer layer of skin?
    (A) First-degree (superficial)
    (B) Second-degree (partial-thickness)
    (C) Third-degree (full-thickness)
    (D) Fourth-degree (deep-thickness)

10. To treat a minor burn, the nursing assistant should
    (A) Use antibacterial ointment
    (B) Use grease, such as butter
    (C) Use ice water
    (D) Use cool, clean water

11. If a resident faints, the nursing assistant should
    (A) Lower the resident to the floor
    (B) Position the resident on his side
    (C) Perform CPR right away
    (D) Help the resident stand up immediately

12. If a resident has a nosebleed, what should be the first step that the nursing assistant takes?
    (A) Report and document the incident.
    (B) Apply pressure consistently until the bleeding stops.
    (C) Apply a cool cloth on the back of the neck, the forehead, or the upper lip.
    (D) Elevate the head of the bed or tell the resident to remain in a sitting position.

13. When a resident is first experiencing signs of insulin reaction, what needs to happen?
    (A) Food that can be rapidly absorbed or a glucose tablet should be consumed.
    (B) The person should lie down and be left alone to rest.
    (C) The nursing assistant should give the resident his diabetes medication.
    (D) CPR measures should be started.

14. Which of the following is true of assisting a resident who is having a seizure?
    (A) The nursing assistant should give the resident water to drink.
    (B) The nursing assistant should hold the resident down if he is shaking severely.
    (C) The nursing assistant should move furniture away to prevent injury to the resident.
    (D) The nursing assistant should open the resident's mouth to move the tongue to the side.

15. Why is a quick response to a suspected stroke/CVA critical?
    (A) A quick response means that the facility will not be liable.
    (B) Early treatment may be able to reduce the severity of the stroke.
    (C) Residents will be able to say their good-byes to family members.
    (D) Residents will experience no side effects at all if there is a quick response.

16. If a resident falls, the nursing assistant should
    (A) Wait until the end of the day to report the fall
    (B) Ask the resident to get up to see if she can walk
    (C) Notify the nurse
    (D) Move the resident to the bed

3. Describe disaster guidelines

Multiple Choice

1. A disaster kit should be assembled before disaster strikes. Disaster supplies include
   (A) A change of clothing
   (B) A television set
   (C) Cosmetics and a hair dryer
   (D) Three pairs of shoes

2. In a disaster, a nursing assistant can stay informed by
   (A) Running out to buy a newspaper
   (B) Calling the fire department
   (C) Listening to instructions from the nurse or administrator
   (D) Texting friends

3. If a disaster is forecast, a nursing assistant can be prepared by
   (A) Powering down her cell phone
   (B) Cleaning her house
   (C) Knowing how to start a fire
   (D) Wearing appropriate clothing and shoes

4. In the event of a tornado, it is best to
   (A) Seek shelter inside, ideally in a steel-framed or concrete building
   (B) Stand flat against the wall next to the windows
   (C) Seek shelter in a mobile home
   (D) Seek shelter outside, ideally in trees or bushes

5. In case of lightning, it is best to
   (A) Find water and stay in the water
   (B) Stand by the largest tree in the area
   (C) Stand close to tall metal objects
   (D) Seek shelter in buildings

6. In case of floods, it is best to
   (A) Fill the bathtub with fresh water
   (B) Drink flood water to stay hydrated
   (C) Put electrical equipment in flood water to avoid fires
   (D) Turn off the gas by yourself

7. In case of earthquakes, it is best to
   (A) Go outside to find the closest tall building
   (B) Stop underneath an overpass if in a car until the shaking stops
   (C) Get under a sturdy piece of furniture
   (D) Stand on a piece of tall furniture to get as high as possible

Emergency Care and Disaster Preparation

8

Human Needs and Human Development

1. Identify basic human needs

Short Answer

1. List five basic physical needs that all humans have.

_____

_____

_____

_____

_____

2. List six psychosocial needs that humans have.

_____

_____

_____

_____

_____

_____

3. Complete your own hierarchy of needs below. Some of the examples have already been completed for you.

Maslow's Hierarchy of Needs

Need

(A) Need for self-actualization

(B) Need for self-esteem

(C) Need for love

(D) Safety and security needs

(E) Physical needs

Example of Need

(A) I need the chance to learn new things.

(B) I need to know that I am doing a good job.

(C) _____

_____

(D) _____

_____

(E) _____

_____

2. Define *holistic care* and explain its importance in health care

Short Answer

1. In your own words, briefly define holistic care.

_____

_____

_____

_____

3. Explain why independence and self-care are important

Fill in the Blank

1. A loss of _____
   is very difficult for a person to deal with.

2. A nursing assistant should allow a resident to do a _____
   independently even if it is easier for the NA to do it.

3. _____ of daily living (ADLs) are personal care tasks a person does every day to care for himself.

4. NAs should encourage _____, regardless of how long it takes or how poorly residents are able to do it.

5. A loss of independence can cause increased _____.

Short Answer

6. Write a brief paragraph explaining everything you did this morning before arriving in class. Include things such as bathing, going to the bathroom, applying makeup, fixing breakfast, brushing your hair, brushing your teeth, reading, walking around your house, etc.

_____

_____

_____

_____

_____

_____

_____

_____

_____

_____

7. How would you feel if you were unable to do one or more of those tasks by yourself?

_____

_____

_____

_____

_____

_____

_____

_____

_____

_____

_____

4. Describe sexual orientation and gender identity and explain ways to accommodate sexual needs

True or False

1. ____ Elderly people no longer have sexual urges.

2. ____ Ability to engage in sexual activity continues unless disease or injury occurs.

3. ____ Residents have the legal right to choose how to express their sexuality.

4. ____ All elderly people have the same sexual behavior and desires.

5. ____ Nursing assistants should assume all residents are heterosexual unless told otherwise.

6. ____ If a person is unable to meet his sexual needs due to a disability, he will no longer have sexual desires.

7. ____ If a resident is physically female but identifies as male, the NA should refer to the resident as "he."

8. ____ People who are confined to wheelchairs cannot have intimate relationships.

9. ____ Lack of privacy is a major reason for lack of sexual expression in long-term care facilities.

10. ____ The nursing assistant should always knock and wait for a response before entering residents' rooms.

11. ____ If a nursing assistant sees a sexual encounter between consenting adult residents, she should ask them to stop and wait until a better time.

12. ____ If a nursing assistant encounters a resident being sexually abused, he should take the resident to a safe place and then notify the nurse.

Matching
Use each letter only once.

13. _____ Bisexual, Bi

14. _____ Cisgender

15. _____ Coming out

16. _____ Cross-dresser

17. _____ Gay

18. _____ Gender identity

19. _____ Heterosexual (straight)

20. _____ Lesbian

21. _____ LGBT

22. _____ LGBTQ

23. _____ Queer

24. _____ Sexual orientation

25. _____ Transgender

26. _____ Transition

(A) Acronym for lesbian, gay, bisexual, transgender, and queer

(B) A person's physical, emotional, and/or romantic attraction to another person

(C) A person whose physical, emotional, and/or romantic attraction is for people of the same sex

(D) A person whose physical, emotional, and/or romantic attraction may be for people of the same gender or a different gender

(E) A continual process of revealing one's sexual orientation or gender identity to others

(F) A deeply felt sense of one's gender

(G) Typically refers to a heterosexual man who sometimes wears clothing and other items associated with women

(H) A person whose gender identity matches his or her birth sex (sex assigned at birth due to anatomy)

(I) A person whose physical, emotional, and/or romantic attraction is for people of the opposite sex

(J) Acronym for lesbian, gay, bisexual, and transgender

(K) A woman whose physical, emotional, and/or romantic attraction is for other women

(L) A person whose gender identity conflicts with his or her birth sex (sex assigned at birth due to anatomy)

(M) The process of changing genders, which can include legal procedures and medical measures

(N) A term used by some people to describe sexual orientation that is not exclusively heterosexual and who feel terms such as lesbian and gay are too limiting

5. Identify ways to help residents meet their spiritual needs

Short Answer
Place a check mark (✓) next to examples of appropriate ways to help residents with their spiritual needs.

1. _____ A resident tells his nursing assistant (NA) that he cannot drink milk with his hamburger due to his religious beliefs. He asks for some water instead. The NA takes the milk away and brings him some water.

2. _____ A resident tells her nursing assistant that she is a Baptist and wants to know when the next Baptist service will be. The NA asks, "Why don't you just attend a Catholic service instead? I'm a Catholic and my church is close by."

3. _____ A resident asks an NA to read a passage from his Bible. The NA opens the Bible and begins to read.

4. _____ A resident wants to see a rabbi. The NA calls the rabbi he wants to see.

5. _____ A nursing assistant sees a Buddha statue in a resident's room. The NA chuckles and tells the resident, "This little guy is so cute."

6. ____ A spiritual leader is visiting with a resident. The NA quietly leaves the room and shuts the door.

7. ____ A resident tells his nursing assistant that he is Muslim. The NA begins to explain Christianity to him and asks him to attend a Christian service just to see what it is like.

8. ____ A resident tells a nursing assistant that she does not believe in God. The NA does believe in God but does not argue with the resident. The NA listens quietly as the resident explains her reasons.

6. Identify ways to accommodate cultural and religious differences

Matching
Use each letter only once.

1. ____ Agnosticism

2. ____ Atheism

3. ____ Buddhism

4. ____ Christianity

5. ____ Hinduism

6. ____ Islam

7. ____ Judaism

(A) Praying fives times a day facing Mecca and worshipping at mosques are part of this religion's practices

(B) Being baptized and receiving communion may be part of this religion's practices

(C) Believing that one does not know or cannot know if God exists

(D) Emphasizing meditation and believing that Nirvana is the highest spiritual plane a person can reach are part of this religion

(E) Believing in karma is part of this religion

(F) Believing that God gave laws through Moses in the form of the Torah is part of this religion

(G) Actively denying the existence of any deity or higher power

Short Answer

8. List three examples of dietary restrictions that may be due to religious beliefs.

_____

_____

_____

_____

_____

_____

_____

_____

Multiple Choice

9. Which of the following is the name of a type of diet in which no animals or animal products are consumed, and animal products may not be used or worn?
(A) High-protein diet
(B) Vegan diet
(C) Kosher diet
(D) Paleo diet

10. Not eating food or eating very little food for a period of time is called
(A) Bingeing
(B) Restricting
(C) Fasting
(D) Purging

7. Describe the need for activity

Crossword

Across

3. A type of cancer that regular physical activity lessens the risk of

5. Type of infection that inactivity can result in

6. The ability to cope with this is one benefit of regular activity

Name: _____

Down

1. Before activities begin, something that NAs assist residents with

2. Something increased by regular activity, in addition to promoting better eating habits

4. Federal law requiring that facilities provide an activities program that meets the interests of residents

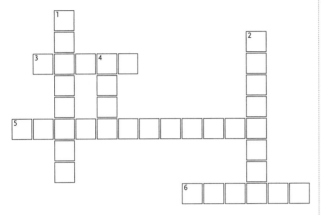

8. Discuss family roles and their significance in health care

Multiple Choice
Read each description below. Choose the term that best defines the type of family that is being described.

1. Mr. Dane's wife died giving birth to their twin girls. Mr. Dane never remarried and raised the girls himself.
   (A) Single-parent family
   (B) Nuclear family
   (C) Blended family
   (D) Extended family

2. Ms. Cone has lived with her best friend, Ms. Lawrence, since they graduated from college together. They both dated men throughout their lives but were never married. Ms. Cone has a teenage daughter who was raised in their household.
   (A) Single-parent family
   (B) Nuclear family
   (C) Blended family
   (D) Extended family

3. Mrs. Rose had three children with her first husband. She divorced him when their youngest child was two years old. Two years later she remarried, and she and her second husband raised her three children as well as one child from his first marriage.
   (A) Single-parent family
   (B) Nuclear family
   (C) Blended family
   (D) Extended family

4. Mrs. Parker was married to her husband for 30 years. They lived together with their two children.
   (A) Single-parent family
   (B) Nuclear family
   (C) Blended family
   (D) Extended family

5. Mr. Potter was married in his twenties. He and his wife moved in with her parents and had three children. Later, when his younger sister was divorced, she also moved in with them.
   (A) Single-parent family
   (B) Nuclear family
   (C) Blended family
   (D) Extended family

6. Mr. Barter and Mr. Singer have been in a committed relationship for 15 years. They live with their 10-year-old daughter.
   (A) Single-parent family
   (B) Nuclear family
   (C) Blended family
   (D) Extended family

7. How is the family of today defined?
   (A) By blood relations
   (B) By how children are raised
   (C) By formal marriages
   (D) By support of one another

9. List ways to respond to emotional needs of residents and their families

True or False

1. _____ If a resident or family member comes to a nursing assistant with a problem or need, the NA should try to empathize.

2. ____ If the NA simply sits quietly and listens when a resident tells her about a problem, the resident will think the NA does not care.

3. ____ Families may seek out nursing assistants because they are the closest staff members to the residents.

4. ____ Nursing assistants should spend all of their time focusing on the residents themselves, not on their families.

5. ____ Using clichés is a good way for NAs to comfort residents.

6. ____ If an NA feels he cannot help a resident, the NA should refer him to another qualified member of the care team.

10. Describe the stages of human growth and development and identify common disorders for each stage

True or False

1. ____ A child takes three years from birth to be able to move around, communicate basic needs, and feed himself.

2. ____ Infant physical development moves from the hands to the head.

3. ____ Caregivers should encourage infants to stand as soon as they can hold their heads up.

4. ____ Putting an infant to sleep on its back can reduce the risk of sudden infant death syndrome (SIDS).

5. ____ Tantrums are common among toddlers.

6. ____ The best way to deal with tantrums is to give the toddler what he wants.

7. ____ Preschool children are too young to know right from wrong.

8. ____ Children learn to speak between the ages of 3 and 6.

9. ____ From the ages of 6 to 10, children learn to get along with each other.

10. ____ School-age children (6 to 10 years) develop cognitively and socially.

11. ____ Preadolescents are often easy to get along with and are able to handle more responsibility than they were before.

12. ____ Puberty is the stage of growth when secondary sex characteristics, such as body hair, appear.

13. ____ Most adolescents do not feel that peer acceptance is important.

14. ____ Adolescents may be moody due to changing hormones and body image concerns.

15. ____ Eating disorders are difficult to deal with but cannot be life-threatening.

16. ____ Due to changes they are experiencing, adolescents may become depressed and may attempt suicide.

17. ____ By 19 years of age, most young adults have stopped developing physically, psychologically, and socially.

18. ____ One developmental task that most young adults undertake is to choose an occupation or career.

19. ____ A "mid-life crisis" is a period of unrest when a person has an unconscious desire for change and fulfillment of unmet goals.

20. ____ Middle-aged adults usually do not experience any physical changes due to aging.

21. ____ Menopause is a condition that occurs in young women when the ovaries begin to secrete hormones.

22. ____ By the time a person reaches late adulthood, he must adjust to the effects of aging.

11. Distinguish between what is true and what is not true about the aging process

True or False

1. ____ Older adults have different capabilities depending upon their health.

2. _____ As people age, they often become lonely, forgetful, and slow.

3. _____ Diseases and illnesses are not normal parts of aging.

4. _____ Many older adults can lead active and healthy lives.

5. _____ Prejudice against older people is as unfounded and unfair as prejudice against racial, ethnic, or religious groups.

6. _____ Television and movies often present an accurate image of what it is like to grow old.

7. _____ Skin becomes drier and less elastic with age.

8. _____ Responses and reflexes quicken as a person ages.

9. _____ Appetite increases with age.

10. _____ Urinary elimination becomes less frequent in older adults.

11. _____ Immunity weakens as a normal part of aging.

12. _____ Depression is normal in the elderly.

13. _____ The loss of ability to think logically is not a normal change of aging.

12. Explain developmental disabilities and list care guidelines

Crossword
Across

2. Intense tantrums, a short attention span, an inability to be empathetic, and an inability to make this type of contact are problems resulting from autism spectrum disorder

4. Split spine

5. Muscle coordination and nerves are affected with this disorder

Down

1. Most common developmental disorder

3. Developmental disability that causes a small skull, flattened nose, and shorter fingers

13. Identify community resources available to help the elderly and people who are developmentally disabled

Short Answer

1. List five community resources available to the elderly.

_____

_____

_____

_____

_____

_____

_____

_____

_____

Name: _____

2. List five community resources to help people who are developmentally disabled.

_____

_____

_____

_____

_____

_____

_____

9

The Healthy Human Body

1. Describe body systems and define key anatomical terms

Matching
Letters may be used more than once.

1. ____ Cells

2. ____ Homeostasis

3. ____ Metabolism

4. ____ Organs

5. ____ Tissues

(A) The body's building blocks

(B) Made up of a group of cells that performs a similar task

(C) The body's physical and chemical processes

(D) Each has a specific function in the body

(E) Condition in which all body systems are working at their best

2. Describe the integumentary system

Fill in the Blank

1. The largest organ and system in the body is the _____.

2. Skin prevents _____ to internal organs.

3. Skin also prevents the loss of too much _____, which is essential to life.

4. The skin is also a _____ organ that feels heat, cold, pain, touch, and pressure.

5. Blood vessels _____, or widen, when the outside temperature is too high.

6. Blood vessels _____, or narrow, when the outside temperature is too cold.

Normal or Sign/Symptom
Determine which of the following is a normal part of the aging process and which is a sign or symptom that needs to be reported to the nurse. Write N for normal aging or S for a sign/symptom to report.

7. ____ Thinning skin

8. ____ Bruises

9. ____ Wounds

10. ____ Wrinkles

11. ____ Brown spots

12. ____ Thinning of fatty tissue

13. ____ Rashes or flaking of skin

14. ____ Thinning hair

15. ____ Less elastic skin

16. ____ Color changes in skin

17. ____ Swelling

18. ____ Drier skin

19. ____ Redness between toes

3. Describe the musculoskeletal system

True or False

1. _____ The body is shaped by muscles, bones, ligaments, tendons, and cartilage.

2. _____ The human body has 215 bones.

3. _____ Bones are made up of dead cells.

4. _____ Bones protect the body's organs.

5. _____ Two bones meet at a joint.

6. _____ A hinge joint, such as the elbow, can bend in two directions.

7. _____ Muscles allow movement of body parts.

8. _____ Skeletal muscles are involuntary muscles.

9. _____ The heart is an involuntary muscle.

10. _____ Range of motion exercises help prevent problems related to immobility.

11. _____ Atrophy occurs when the muscle weakens, decreases in size, and wastes away.

12. _____ One way to prevent falls is to keep walkers or canes within reach.

Normal or Sign/Symptom

13. _____ Bruising

14. _____ Weakening of muscles

15. _____ Loss of muscle tone

16. _____ Change in ability to do routine movements

17. _____ Loss of bone density

18. _____ Increased brittleness of bones

19. _____ Aches and pains

20. _____ Loss of height

21. _____ Pain during movement

22. _____ Increased swelling of joints

23. _____ White, shiny, warm, or red areas over a joint

24. _____ Slowing of body movement

4. Describe the nervous system

Multiple Choice

1. The nervous system
   (A) Gives the body shape and structure
   (B) Controls and coordinates body functions
   (C) Is the largest organ in the body
   (D) Pumps blood through the blood vessels to the cells

2. The basic unit of the nervous system is the
   (A) Neuron
   (B) Message
   (C) Brain
   (D) Spinal cord

3. The two main parts of the nervous system are
   (A) The cardiovascular system and integumentary system
   (B) Neurons and receptors
   (C) The body and the brain
   (D) The central nervous system and peripheral nervous system

4. The central nervous system (CNS) is made up of
   (A) The brain and spinal cord
   (B) Muscles and bones
   (C) Neurons and receptors
   (D) The heart and lungs

5. The peripheral nervous system (PNS) deals with the outer part of the body via the
   (A) Brain
   (B) Cerebrum
   (C) Nerves
   (D) Right hemisphere

6. What cushions the brain and spinal cord against injury?
   (A) The nerves
   (B) The spinal column
   (C) The brainstem
   (D) Cerebrospinal fluid

7. The _____ is the part of the brain that controls thinking, speech, and voluntary muscles.
   (A) Brainstem
   (B) Cerebellum
   (C) Cerebral cortex
   (D) Right hemisphere

8. The left hemisphere of the brain controls
   (A) The left side of the body
   (B) The right side of the body
   (C) Both sides of the body
   (D) Memory

9. The brainstem controls
   (A) Smooth movements
   (B) Breathing and swallowing
   (C) Jerky movements
   (D) Emotions

10. The nerve pathways in the spinal cord conduct messages between
    (A) The heart and the blood
    (B) The cerebrum and cerebellum
    (C) The brain and the body
    (D) The muscles and the bones

Normal or Sign/Symptom

11. _____ Inability to move one side of the body

12. _____ Depression or mood changes

13. _____ Fatigue or pain with movement

14. _____ Shaking

15. _____ Decreased sense of heat and cold

16. _____ Slurring of speech

17. _____ Decreased ability to perform ADLs

18. _____ Slower reflexes

19. _____ Trouble swallowing

20. _____ Confusion

21. _____ Decreased sensitivity of nerve endings in skin

22. _____ Violent behavior

23. _____ Minor short-term memory loss

24. _____ Changes in vision

Short Answer

Sense Organs

25. List the five sense organs of the body.

   _____

   _____

   _____

   _____

   _____

26. Which part of the eye sends a message to the brain so that a person can see?

   _____

   _____

   _____

   _____

27. List the three parts of the ear.

   _____

   _____

   _____

5. Describe the circulatory system

Multiple Choice

1. What functions as the pump of the circulatory system?
   (A) Heart
   (B) Lungs
   (C) Lymph
   (D) Blood

2. How many chambers does the heart have?
   (A) Two
   (B) Three
   (C) Four
   (D) Five

3. The contracting phase of the heart, when the ventricles pump blood through the blood vessels, is called
   (A) Capillary
   (B) Systole
   (C) Diastole
   (D) Blood exchange

4. The resting phase of the heart, when the chambers fill with blood, is called
    (A) Capillary
    (B) Systole
    (C) Diastole
    (D) Blood exchange

5. What gives blood its red color?
    (A) Plasma
    (B) Iron
    (C) Lymph
    (D) Glucose

6. What is plasma mostly made up of?
    (A) Water
    (B) Oxygen
    (C) Lymph
    (D) Minerals

Normal or Sign/Symptom

7. ____ Severe headache

8. ____ Heart pumps less efficiently

9. ____ Chest pain

10. ____ Swelling of hands or feet

11. ____ Changes in pulse rate

12. ____ Bluish hands or feet

13. ____ Fatigue

14. ____ Shortness of breath

6. Describe the respiratory system

True or False

1. ____ Respiration occurs in the lungs.

2. ____ Expiration is breathing in.

3. ____ The respiratory system brings oxygen into the body and removes carbon dioxide.

4. ____ The larynx is also called the windpipe.

5. ____ Oxygen and carbon dioxide are exchanged between the alveoli and the capillaries.

6. ____ The pleura is a membrane that covers the lungs.

7. ____ Regular exercise and movement should be encouraged.

Normal or Sign/Symptom

8. ____ Decreased lung strength and capacity

9. ____ Discolored sputum

10. ____ Need to sit after mild exertion

11. ____ Shallow breathing

12. ____ Bluish legs

13. ____ Weaker voice

14. ____ Coughing

15. ____ Nasal congestion

16. ____ Change in respiratory rate

7. Describe the urinary system

Short Answer

1. List the two vital functions of the urinary system.

    _____

    _____

    _____

    _____

    _____

2. What is one reason why the female bladder is more likely to become infected by bacteria than the male bladder?

    _____

    _____

    _____

    _____

Normal or Sign/Symptom

3. ____ Pain during urination

4. ____ Bladder does not empty completely

5. ____ Bladder feels full or painful

6. ____ Pain in kidney region

7. ____ Changes in color of urine

8. ____ Urinary incontinence

9. ____ Inadequate fluid intake

8. Describe the gastrointestinal system

Crossword

Across

3. The process of expelling wastes (made up of the waste products of food and fluids) that are not absorbed into the cells

4. Involuntary contractions that move food into the stomach from the esophagus

6. The transfer of nutrients from the intestines to the cells

7. Semi-solid material made up of water, solid waste material, bacteria, and mucus that passes through the rectum and out of the body

Down

1. The process of preparing food physically and chemically so that it can be absorbed into the cells

2. Semi-liquid substance created by the breaking down of food in the stomach

5. Muscular pouch located in the upper left part of the abdominal cavity

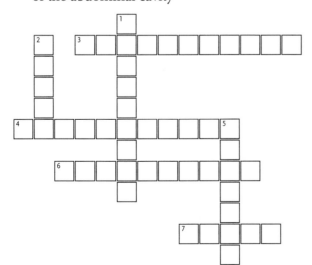

Normal or Sign/Symptom

8. ____ Flatulence

9. ____ Decreased saliva

10. ____ Poor appetite

11. ____ Black stool

12. ____ Fecal incontinence

13. ____ Decreased absorption of nutrients

14. ____ Diarrhea

15. ____ Less efficient digestion

16. ____ Heartburn

9. Describe the endocrine system

Matching
Use each letter only once.

1. ____ Adrenal glands

2. ____ Antidiuretic hormone

3. ____ Gonads

4. ____ Insulin

5. ____ Oxytocin

6. ____ Pancreas

7. ____ Parathyroid glands

8. ____ Pituitary gland

9. ____ Thyroid gland

(A) Secretes insulin

(B) Produces hormones that regulate salt and water absorption in kidneys and produce the hormone adrenaline

(C) Located in the neck in front of the larynx and produces thyroid hormone

(D) Master gland of the body

(E) Secretes a hormone to regulate calcium use

(F) Moves glucose from the blood into the cells for energy for the body

(G) Controls the balance of fluids in the body

(H) Causes the uterus to contract during and after childbirth

(I) Produces hormones that regulate the ability to reproduce

Normal or Sign/Symptom

10. ____ Excessive perspiration

11. ____ Dizziness

12. ____ Hyperactivity

13. ____ Blurred vision

14. ____ Decreased ability to handle stress

15. ____ Irritability

16. ____ Headache

17. ____ Reduced insulin production

18. ____ Hunger

19. ____ Decrease in progesterone levels

20. ____ Confusion

21. ____ Weakness

10. Describe the reproductive system

Multiple Choice

1. The reproductive system allows humans to
   (A) Move and speak
   (B) Create human life
   (C) Think logically
   (D) Fight disease

2. The hormone needed for male reproductive organs to function properly is
   (A) Sperm
   (B) Adrenaline
   (C) Estrogen
   (D) Testosterone

3. The male and female sex glands are the
   (A) Glands
   (B) Ureters
   (C) Gonads
   (D) Urethras

4. The tube through which males pass both urine and semen is called the
   (A) Prostate
   (B) Penis
   (C) Urethra
   (D) Seminal vesicle

5. The gonads in human females are called
   (A) Ovaries
   (B) Eggs
   (C) Testicles
   (D) Sex cells

6. The female reproductive cycle is maintained by the hormones
   (A) Estrogen and progesterone
   (B) Adrenaline and progesterone
   (C) Testosterone and ADH
   (D) Insulin and testosterone

7. The _____ contains blood vessels to provide for the growth of an embryo.
   (A) Endometrium
   (B) Uterus
   (C) Fallopian tube
   (D) Fundus

8. A fetus develops inside the
   (A) Endometrium
   (B) Cervix
   (C) Fallopian tube
   (D) Fundus

Normal or Sign/Symptom

9. ____ Erectile dysfunction

10. ____ Decrease in estrogen

11. ____ Swelling of genitals

12. ____ Enlarged prostate gland

13. ____ Menopause

14. ____ Discharge from penis

15. ____ Blood in stool

16. ____ Painful intercourse

17. ____ Decrease in sperm production

18. ____ Sores on genitals

19. ____ Difficulty with urination

11. Describe the immune and lymphatic systems

Short Answer

1. What is the difference between nonspecific immunity and specific immunity?

_____

_____

_____

_____

_____

_____

_____

2. What two systems are related to the lymphatic system?

_____

_____

_____

_____

_____

3. How is lymph fluid circulated?

_____

_____

_____

_____

_____

Normal or Sign/Symptom

4. _____ Swelling of lymph nodes

5. _____ Increased fatigue

6. _____ Decreased response to vaccines

7. _____ Increased risk of infection

The Healthy Human Body

10

Positioning, Transfers, and Ambulation

1. Review the principles of body mechanics

Fill in the Blank

1. _____ the load.

2. Think ahead, _____,
   and communicate the move.

3. Check your base of
   _____.
   Be sure you have firm
   _____.

4. _____ what you are
   lifting.

5. Keep your back
   _____.

6. Begin in a squatting position and lift with
   your _____.

7. _____
   your stomach muscles when beginning the
   lift.

8. Keep the object
   _____
   to your body.

9. _____
   when possible rather than lifting.

2. Explain positioning and describe how to safely position residents

Labeling
Label each position that is illustrated below and describe appropriate comfort measures for each.

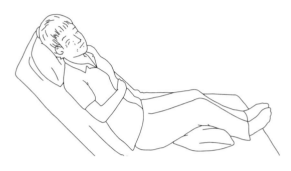

1. _____

Comfort measures: _____

_____

_____

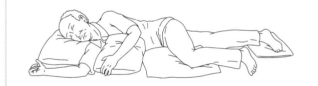

2. _____

Comfort measures: _____

_____

_____

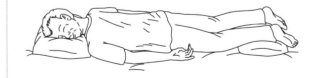

3. _____

Comfort measures: _____

_____

_____

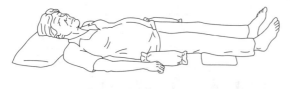

4. _____

Comfort measures: _____

_____

_____

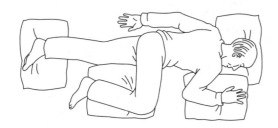

5. _____

Comfort measures: _____

_____

_____

Multiple Choice

6. Why do residents who spend a lot of time in beds or wheelchairs need to be repositioned often?
    (A) Repositioning helps prevent boredom.
    (B) They are at risk of skin breakdown and pressure injuries.
    (C) Staff need to make sure residents are awakened regularly.
    (D) Their family members will often sue the facility if they are not.

7. In this position the resident is lying on either side:
    (A) Supine
    (B) Lateral
    (C) Prone
    (D) Fowler's

8. In this position, the resident is lying on his stomach:
    (A) Sims'
    (B) Lateral
    (C) Prone
    (D) Fowler's

9. A draw sheet is used to
    (A) Make changing the bottom bed sheet easier
    (B) Help residents sleep better
    (C) Reposition residents without causing shearing
    (D) Prevent incontinence

10. Logrolling is
    (A) A way to measure the weight of a resident who is bedbound
    (B) One way to record vital signs for a resident who cannot get out of bed easily
    (C) Moving a resident as a unit without disturbing alignment
    (D) A special method of bedmaking

11. Dangling is
    (A) Lying in the supine position
    (B) Doing a few sit-ups in bed to get used to the upright position
    (C) Elevating the resident's feet with pillows
    (D) A way to help residents regain balance before standing up

12. A resident in the Fowler's position is
    (A) In a semi-sitting position
    (B) Lying flat on his back
    (C) In a left side-lying position
    (D) Lying on his stomach

3. Describe how to safely transfer residents

Multiple Choice

1. Which of the following statements is true of working with residents in wheelchairs?
    (A) Before transferring a resident, the NA should make sure the wheelchair is unlocked and movable.
    (B) The NA should check the resident's alignment in the chair after a transfer is complete.
    (C) To fold a standard wheelchair, the NA should turn it upside-down to make the seat flatten.
    (D) All residents will need their NAs to transfer them to their wheelchairs.

2. Some residents have a side of the body that is weaker than the other one. The weaker side of the body should be referred to as the
   (A) Released side
   (B) Separated side
   (C) Ambulated side
   (D) Involved side

3. When applying a transfer belt, the nursing assistant should place it
   (A) Around the wheelchair's backrest
   (B) Underneath the resident's clothing, on bare skin
   (C) Over the resident's clothing and around the waist
   (D) Around the nursing assistant's waist so the resident can hold on to it

4. The following piece of equipment may be used to help transfer residents who are unable to bear weight on their legs:
   (A) Sling
   (B) Slide board
   (C) Wheeled table
   (D) Folded blanket

5. Which of the following statements is true of using mechanical, or hydraulic, lifts to assist with transfers?
   (A) When doing this type of transfer, it is safer for one person to transfer the resident by himself.
   (B) The legs of the stand need to be closed, in their narrowest position, before helping the resident into the lift.
   (C) Lifts help prevent injury to the nursing assistant and the resident.
   (D) It is best to use mechanical lifts when moving the resident a long distance.

6. When transferring residents who have one-sided weakness, which side moves first?
   (A) Left side
   (B) Either side
   (C) Weaker side
   (D) Stronger side

7. If a resident starts to fall during the transfer, the best response by the nursing assistant would be to
   (A) Bend her knees and lower the resident to the floor
   (B) Catch the resident under the arms to stop the fall
   (C) Move away and allow the resident to fall on her own
   (D) Have the resident fall on top of her to break the fall

4. Discuss how to safely ambulate residents

Multiple Choice

1. A resident who has some difficulty with balance but can bear weight on both legs should use a
   (A) Walker
   (B) Crutch
   (C) Wheelchair
   (D) Transfer board

2. Ambulation is another word for
   (A) Walking
   (B) Movement in a wheelchair
   (C) Riding in an ambulance
   (D) Logrolling

3. In addition to a gait belt, what equipment should the nursing assistant have when assisting a resident to ambulate?
   (A) Mechanical lift
   (B) Rocking chair
   (C) Extra pillows
   (D) Nonskid shoes

4. If the resident is unable to stand without help, the nursing assistant should
   (A) Hold the resident close to the NA's center of gravity
   (B) Tell the resident to stand on the count of three
   (C) Brace the resident's lower extremities
   (D) Adjust the bed to its highest position

5. When helping a resident who is visually impaired to walk, it is important for the nursing assistant to
   (A) Keep the resident in front of her
   (B) Let the resident walk beside and slightly behind her
   (C) Walk quickly
   (D) Avoid mentioning stepping up or down

6. Which of the following assistive devices for walking has four rubber-tipped feet?
   (A) C cane
   (B) Quad cane
   (C) Crutch
   (D) Gait belt

7. When using a cane, the resident should place it on his _____ side.
   (A) Left
   (B) Right
   (C) Weaker
   (D) Stronger

11

Admitting, Transferring, and Discharging

1. Describe how residents may feel when entering a facility

Short Answer

1. What makes moving to a long-term care facility (LTCF) a big adjustment for new residents?

    _____
    _____
    _____
    _____
    _____
    _____
    _____
    _____
    _____
    _____
    _____
    _____
    _____

2. Why might lesbian, gay, bisexual, transgender, or queer (LGBTQ) residents have additional concerns when moving into a care facility?

    _____
    _____
    _____
    _____

_____
_____
_____

2. Explain the nursing assistant's role in the admission process

Fill in the Blank

1. _____ is often the first time a nursing assistant meets a new resident.

2. The NA should try to make sure the resident has a positive _____ of her and her facility.

3. The NA should prepare the _____ before the resident arrives.

4. The NA should ask _____ to find out a resident's personal preferences and _____.

5. The NA should _____ herself to the resident and state her position.

6. The NA should always call a resident by her _____ name until she tells the NA what she prefers to be called.

7. The NA should try to make sure the new resident feels welcome and wanted. The NA should not _____ the process or the new resident.

8. The NA can help the resident by explaining daily life in the facility and offering to take the resident on a _____.

Name: _____

9. New residents must be given a copy of their legal _____.

10. It is important for the nursing assistant to _____ the new resident's condition in order to recognize any changes that may take place later.

11. A resident has a legal right to have his _____ items that he has brought with him treated carefully.

Short Answer

12. Why must a nursing assistant report any weight a resident loses?

_____
_____
_____
_____
_____
_____

13. How many inches are in one foot?

_____

Labeling

Looking at each of the readings shown below, determine each resident's weight for numbers 14 to 17 and height for numbers 18 to 21.

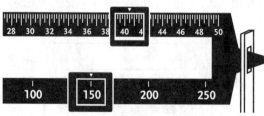

14. _____

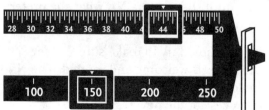

15. _____

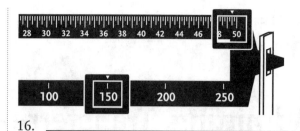

16. _____

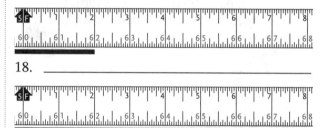

17. _____

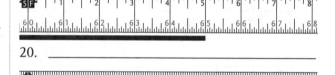

18. _____

19. _____

20. _____

21. _____

3. Explain the nursing assistant's role during an in-house transfer of a resident

True or False

1. _____ A transfer to a new facility or hospital is normally easy for residents to handle.

2. _____ Residents should be informed of transfers as early as possible.

3. _____ The resident will usually pack her own belongings for a transfer.

4. _____ The nursing assistant should introduce the resident to everyone in the new area.

5. ____ One way that a nursing assistant can involve the resident with the packing process is to show the resident her empty closet.

4. Explain the nursing assistant's role in the discharge of a resident

Scenario

1. Mr. Carpenter has been at the Green Garden Skilled Nursing Facility for six months to recover from a broken hip. He has made an excellent recovery. His doctor has written a discharge order, and he is now ready to return home. As the nursing assistant is packing his things for him, Mr. Carpenter tells her that he is afraid that he will not be able to take care of himself at home. What can the NA say to express concern and reassure him?

_____

_____

_____

_____

2. What are five things that the nurse will probably discuss with Mr. Carpenter and his family before he is discharged?

_____

_____

_____

_____

_____

3. What is a responsibility of the nursing assistant regarding a resident's discharge?

_____

_____

_____

_____

_____

_____

5. Describe the nursing assistant's role in physical exams

Multiple Choice

1. What are the nursing assistant's duties during residents' physical exams?
   (A) Performing the exams
   (B) Giving injections
   (C) Making recommendations for treatment
   (D) Gathering equipment for the doctor

2. In which position is the resident placed for examination of the breasts, chest, abdomen, and perineal area?
   (A) Dorsal recumbent position
   (B) Lithotomy position
   (C) Knee-chest position
   (D) Trendelenburg position

3. Which of the following pieces of equipment is used to measure blood pressure?
   (A) Reflex hammer
   (B) Thermometer
   (C) Sphygmomanometer
   (D) Otoscope

4. In which position is the resident in stirrups in order to examine the vagina?
   (A) Sims' position
   (B) Lithotomy position
   (C) Knee-chest position
   (D) Prone position

5. In which position is the resident on her abdomen with her knees pulled toward the abdomen in order to examine the rectum or the vagina?
   (A) Lateral position
   (B) Lithotomy position
   (C) Knee-chest position
   (D) Prone position

Short Answer

6. List three responsibilities of a nursing assistant after a resident's physical exam has been completed.

_____

Admitting, Transferring, and Discharging

_____

_____

_____

_____

_____

_____

_____

_____

_____

7. List two legal rights that residents are entitled to regarding exams.

_____

_____

_____

_____

_____

_____

_____

12

The Resident's Unit

1. Explain why a comfortable environment is important for the resident's well-being

Fill in the Blank

1. Common _____ in facilities can upset and/or irritate residents.

2. Nursing assistants should not _____ equipment or meal trays.

3. It is a good idea for an NA to keep her _____ low and to _____ doors when residents ask her to.

4. To control odors, an NA should clean up after episodes of _____ and change incontinence _____ as soon as they are soiled.

5. The NA should empty and clean bedpans, _____, commodes, and _____ basins right away.

6. Giving regular oral care and _____ care can help avoid body and breath odors.

7. Due to loss of protective fatty tissue and illness, older residents may feel _____ often.

8. To help residents stay comfortable, the NA should _____ clothes and bed covers for warmth and keep residents _____ during personal care.

9. Adequate _____ promotes safety and helps prevent falls. Residents may prefer _____ rooms when they are ill or are sleeping.

2. Describe a standard resident unit

True or False

1. ____ A resident's room is his home and must be treated with respect.

2. ____ It is never necessary for a nursing assistant to knock and wait for permission to enter a resident's room.

3. ____ Normally residents' beds are kept in their highest position, which reduces the risk of falls.

4. ____ Emesis basins and soap may be stored inside the bedside stand.

5. ____ Urinals and bedpans are normally stored on top of the overbed table.

6. ____ Call lights must always be answered promptly.

7. ____ Call lights should be placed wherever it is easiest for the nursing assistant to reach them.

8. ____ Privacy curtains block sight, as well as sound.

9. ____ Residents have a legal right to have their privacy protected when receiving care.

10. ____ Soiled linen should be placed on the overbed table when changing a resident's bed.

3. Discuss how to care for and clean unit equipment

Multiple Choice

1. If a nursing assistant is asked to use a piece of equipment he does not know how to use, he should
   (A) Figure it out as he goes along
   (B) Try to perform the procedure without using the equipment
   (C) Ask for help
   (D) Refuse to use the equipment

2. Disposable equipment is
   (A) Used once and then discarded
   (B) Used three times and then discarded
   (C) Sterilized before it is reused
   (D) Disinfected after each use

3. Which of the following is an example of disposable equipment?
   (A) Bedpan
   (B) Stethoscope
   (C) Gloves
   (D) Blood pressure cuff

4. Call lights should be placed
   (A) Next to the television
   (B) On the overbed table
   (C) Near the door
   (D) Within the resident's reach

4. Explain the importance of sleep and factors affecting sleep

Short Answer

1. List five things that can disrupt a resident's sleep.

   _____

   _____

   _____

   _____

   _____

   _____

   _____

2. List four things that staff should observe for when a resident complains that she is not sleeping well.

   _____

   _____

   _____

   _____

   _____

   _____

   _____

   _____

5. Describe bedmaking guidelines and perform proper bedmaking

Multiple Choice

1. Why is it important for nursing assistants to change bed linen often?
   (A) To get residents out of bed and moving around
   (B) To rotate clean sheets evenly
   (C) To keep NAs' skills up-to-date
   (D) To prevent infection and to promote comfort

2. Why should bed linen be carried away from the nursing assistant's body?
   (A) To prevent contamination of clothing
   (B) To keep the linen neat
   (C) To avoid mixing up the linen from different residents
   (D) For proper body alignment

3. When removing dirty linen, the NA should
   (A) Fold it so that the soiled area is outside
   (B) Roll it so that the soiled area is inside
   (C) Gather it in a bunch
   (D) Shake it to remove particles

4. When a resident cannot get out of bed
   (A) The bed cannot be changed
   (B) The resident will be moved to a stretcher for bed changing
   (C) The nurse will change the bed
   (D) The bed should be raised to a safe height before making it

5. Soiled linen should be bagged
    (A) In the hallway
    (B) In another resident's room
    (C) At the point of origin
    (D) At the nurses' station

6. A surgical bed is
    (A) A bed used during surgery
    (B) A bed made to easily accept residents
        returning on stretchers
    (C) A bed used for special personal care
        procedures
    (D) Any bed on a residential unit

7. A bed made with the bedspread and blankets
    in place is called a(n)
    (A) Open bed
    (B) Stretcher bed
    (C) Closed bed
    (D) Completed bed

Name: _____

13

Personal Care Skills

1. Explain personal care of residents

True or False

1. _____ Promoting independence is part of a nursing assistant's care of residents.

2. _____ Styling one's hair is part of grooming oneself.

3. _____ Perineal care is care of the fingernails and toenails.

4. _____ It is best for the nursing assistant to make decisions about when and where procedures will be done.

5. _____ Having care explained before it is performed is a resident's legal right.

6. _____ The nursing assistant should knock and wait for permission to enter a resident's room.

7. _____ Personal care provides the nursing assistant with an opportunity to observe a resident's mental state.

8. _____ If a resident appears tired during a procedure, the nursing assistant should encourage him to keep going so that the procedure is more efficient.

9. _____ Before leaving a resident's room, the nursing assistant should leave the bed in its highest positions.

10. _____ The call light should always be left where the nursing assistant can easily reach it when she returns to the room.

2. Identify guidelines for providing skin care and preventing pressure injuries

Crossword

Across

2. The bottom sheet on a resident's bed must be kept tight and free from _____.

5. Cloth-covered items that keep the hand or fingers in a normal, natural position

6. A problem that can result from pulling a resident across the sheet when transferring him

8. Skin should be kept clean and ____.

Down

1. Keeps covers from resting on the legs and feet

3. One type of material that prevents air from circulating, causing the skin to sweat

4. At a minimum, the number of hours at which immobile residents should be repositioned

7. Skin this color should not be massaged

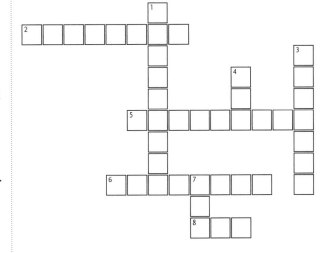

Personal Care Skills

Labeling

For each position shown, list the areas at risk for pressure injuries.

Lateral Position

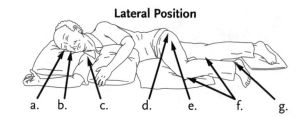

a.   b.   c.   d.   e.   f.   g.

9. Lateral Position

a. _____
b. _____
c. _____
d. _____
e. _____
f. _____
g. _____

Prone Position

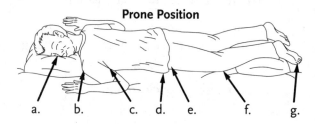

a.   b.   c.   d.   e.   f.   g.

10. Prone Position

a. _____
b. _____
c. _____
d. _____
e. _____
f. _____
g. _____

Supine Position

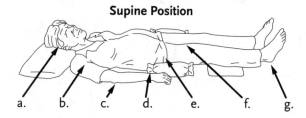

a.   b.   c.   d.   e.   f.   g.

11. Supine Position

a. _____
b. _____
c. _____
d. _____
e. _____
f. _____
g. _____

True or False

12. ____ With a stage 1 pressure injury, skin is intact but may appear red and may be warmer than the area around it.

13. ____ Immobile residents should be repositioned every four hours.

14. ____ Areas of the body where bone is close to the skin are at a higher risk for skin breakdown.

15. ____ Residents seated in wheelchairs do not need to be repositioned.

16. ____ The nursing assistant should massage any red areas he notices.

17. ____ Proper nutrition helps keep the skin healthy.

18. ____ When transferring or positioning residents, pull them across the sheets to make the job easier.

19. ____ Another name for pressure injuries is decubitus ulcers.

20. ____ Common sites for pressure injuries are the chest, nose, and hands.

21. ____ A type of device that helps support and align a limb is called an orthosis.

3. Explain guidelines for assisting with bathing

Multiple Choice

1. A partial bath includes washing a resident's
    (A) Feet
    (B) Genitals
    (C) Legs
    (D) Back

2. Which of the following should be used to wash the resident's face when giving a bed bath?
    (A) Washcloth and water
    (B) Washcloth and soap
    (C) Brush and soap
    (D) Washcloth and moisturizing cream

3. Who is best able to choose a comfortable water temperature for the resident?
    (A) The nursing assistant
    (B) The resident
    (C) The resident's family
    (D) The nurse

4. How hot should the water be when shampooing a resident's hair?
    (A) No higher than 105°F
    (B) No higher than 110°F
    (C) No higher than 115°F
    (D) No higher than 120°F

5. The resident's perineum should be washed
    (A) Twice a day
    (B) Once a day
    (C) Once a week
    (D) Every other day

6. Which of the following products should be used when giving a shower or tub bath?
    (A) Baby powder
    (B) Body oil
    (C) Shampoo
    (D) Talcum powder

7. When should gloves be changed during a bed bath?
    (A) Before washing the perineal area
    (B) Before washing the arms and axillae
    (C) Before washing the hands
    (D) Before washing the abdomen

4. Explain guidelines for assisting with grooming

Short Answer

1. List one benefit of regular grooming.

    _____

    _____

    _____

    _____

2. Describe two grooming routines that are important in your life. Why do you think routines are important to people even when they are ill?

3. What is one reason why careful foot care is important?

    _____

    _____

    _____

    _____

    _____

    _____

4. Where on the foot should a nursing assistant not apply lotion when giving foot care?

    _____

    _____

    _____

    _____

    _____

5. Why should a nursing assistant wear gloves while shaving a resident?

    _____

    _____

    _____

    _____

6. Why should electric razors not be used near any water or when oxygen is in use?

_____

_____

_____

_____

_____

_____

7. The textbook states, "Residents' hair should never be combed or brushed into childish styles." Why do you think this statement is included?

_____

_____

_____

_____

_____

_____

8. What are ways to prevent the spread of lice?

_____

_____

_____

_____

_____

5. List guidelines for assisting with dressing

Multiple Choice

1. Which of the following would be the best type of clothing for a resident to wear during the day?
   (A) A comfortable nightgown
   (B) A clean blouse and pair of pants
   (C) A flannel pajama top and bottoms
   (D) A bathrobe and slippers

2. For a resident who has weakness or paralysis on one side, the nursing assistant should place the _____ arm or leg through the garment first.
   (A) Stronger
   (B) Weaker
   (C) Right
   (D) Left

3. When undressing a resident who has weakness or paralysis on one side, the nursing assistant should start with the _____ side.
   (A) Stronger
   (B) Weaker
   (C) Right
   (D) Left

4. The resident's clothing for the day should be chosen by the
   (A) Resident
   (B) Resident's friend
   (C) Nursing assistant
   (D) Physical therapist

6. Identify guidelines for proper oral care

Short Answer

1. How often should oral care be performed? When should it be done?

_____

_____

_____

_____

_____

_____

_____

2. List eight signs to observe and report when performing oral care.

_____

_____

_____

_____

_____

_____

_____

_____

_____

_____

_____

_____

3. What is aspiration? How can the nursing assistant help prevent aspiration during oral care of unconscious residents?

_____

_____

_____

_____

_____

_____

_____

7. Define *dentures* and explain how to care for dentures

Multiple Choice

1. Dentures must be handled carefully because
    (A) A resident cannot eat without them
    (B) They do not cost much
    (C) A resident will look unattractive without them
    (D) They are sharp

2. Dentures should be cleaned by
    (A) Using soapy water and a denture brush
    (B) Using cool water and denture cleanser
    (C) Soaking them in hot water before scrubbing them
    (D) Using rubbing alcohol and a toothbrush

3. How should dentures be stored?
    (A) In a denture cup
    (B) In ice water
    (C) Wrapped in a paper towel
    (D) In hot water

4. If the nursing assistant is removing a resident's dentures, the resident should be
    (A) Lying down on his back
    (B) Standing
    (C) Sitting upright
    (D) Lying down on his side

5. When inserting dentures, the nursing assistant should
    (A) Apply antibiotic ointment to the dentures first
    (B) Use her bare hands for a better grip
    (C) Use tongs to get the dentures to stick
    (D) Place upper denture into the mouth by turning it at an angle

Personal Care Skills

Personal Care Skills

14

Basic Nursing Skills

1. Explain the importance of monitoring vital signs

Short Answer

1. What might changes in vital signs indicate?

_____

_____

_____

_____

2. Which changes should be immediately reported to the nurse?

_____

_____

_____

_____

_____

_____

2. List guidelines for measuring body temperature

Short Answer

1. What are five sites for measuring body temperature?

_____

_____

_____

_____

2. Name seven conditions that indicate a person's temperature should not be taken orally.

_____

_____

_____

_____

_____

_____

_____

_____

_____

Labeling
For each of the illustrations of thermometers shown below, write the temperature reading to the nearest tenth degree in the blank provided.

3. _____

4. _____

5. _____

6. _____

7. _____

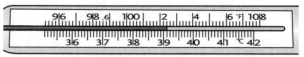

8. _____

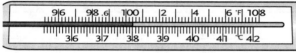

9. _____

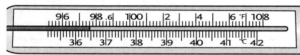

10. _____

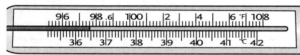

11. _____

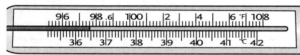

12. _____

Multiple Choice

13. A rectal thermometer is usually color-coded
    (A) Green or blue
    (B) Red or orange
    (C) Black or white
    (D) White or yellow

14. Which of the following thermometers is used once and then discarded?
    (A) Oral thermometer
    (B) Rectal thermometer
    (C) Disposable thermometer
    (D) Tympanic thermometer

15. Which of the following temperature sites is another word for the armpit area?
    (A) Oral
    (B) Rectal
    (C) Axilla
    (D) Tympanic

16. Which temperature site is considered to be the most accurate?
    (A) Mouth
    (B) Rectum
    (C) Temporal artery
    (D) Ear

17. How long do digital thermometers take to display a person's temperature?
    (A) 2 to 60 seconds
    (B) 1 to 2 minutes
    (C) 3 minutes
    (D) Less than 1 second

18. How are temporal artery thermometers used to measure body temperature?
    (A) The thermometer is inserted into the person's mouth and under the tongue for approximately one minute.
    (B) The thermometer is scanned across the forehead.
    (C) The thermometer is placed in the axillary area for eight to 10 minutes.
    (D) The thermometer is inserted 1/4 inch into the ear.

3. List guidelines for measuring pulse and respirations

Multiple Choice

1. Where is the apical pulse located?
   (A) Underneath a person's chin
   (B) On the inside of the wrist
   (C) On the inside of the elbow
   (D) On the left side of the chest, just below the nipple

2. Which pulse is most often used for measuring pulse rate?
   (A) Apical pulse
   (B) Femoral pulse
   (C) Pedal pulse
   (D) Radial pulse

3. The medical term for difficulty breathing is
   (A) Dyspeptic
   (B) Dysphagia
   (C) Dyspnea
   (D) Diastolic

4. Which of the following is an instrument that can listen to sounds within the body?
   (A) Reflex hammer
   (B) Scalpel
   (C) Stethoscope
   (D) Microscope

5. Inhaling air into the lungs is also called
   (A) Inspiration
   (B) Expiration
   (C) Rhythm
   (D) Pulse

6. Exhaling air out of the lungs is also called
   (A) Inspiration
   (B) Expiration
   (C) Rhythm
   (D) Pulse

7. The normal respiration rate for adults ranges from
   (A) 5 to 10 breaths per minute
   (B) 12 to 20 breaths per minute
   (C) 25 to 32 breaths per minute
   (D) 7 to 11 breaths per minute

8. Why is it important for the nursing assistant to observe respirations without letting the resident know what she is doing?
   (A) People may breathe more quickly if they know they are being observed.
   (B) People will hold their breath if they know what an NA wants to measure.
   (C) The procedure takes less time if the resident is unaware of what is happening.
   (D) Observing respirations is a painful process for most people.

4. Explain guidelines for measuring blood pressure

Matching
Use each letter only once.

1. _____ Diastolic phase

2. _____ Hypertension

3. _____ Hypotension

4. _____ mmHg

5. _____ Sphygmomanometer

6. _____ Systolic phase

(A) Blood pressure measurement that reflects the phase when the heart is at work

(B) Medical term for low blood pressure

(C) Blood pressure measurement that reflects the phase when the heart relaxes

(D) Medical term for high blood pressure

(E) Device that measures blood pressure

(F) Abbreviation for millimeters of mercury

Short Answer
For each of the gauges shown below, record the blood pressure shown and answer the question.

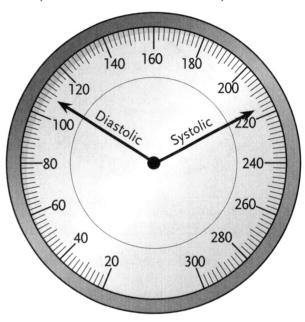

7. _____
   Is this reading within normal range?

   _____

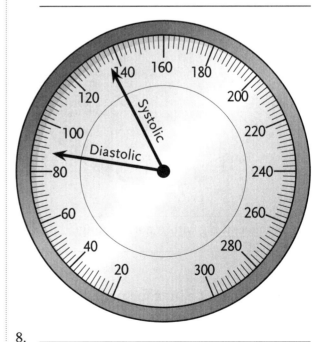

8. _____
   Is this reading within normal range?

   _____

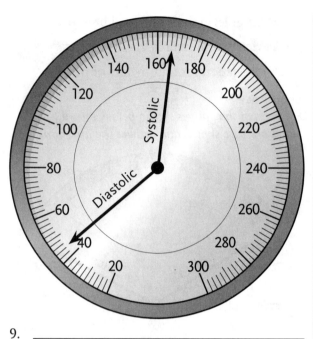

9. _____
   Is this reading within normal range?
   _____

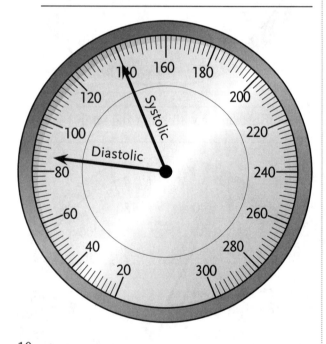

10. _____
    Is this reading within normal range?
    _____

5. Describe guidelines for pain management

Short Answer

1. If a resident complains of pain, what questions should the nursing assistant ask to get the most accurate information?

2. What are barriers to managing pain?

6. Explain the benefits of warm and cold applications

Crossword
Across

3. One benefit of cold applications is that they can bring this down

4. Type of application that helps stop bleeding

6. A warm soak of the perineal area to clean perineal wounds and reduce pain

Down

1. A condition that could cause a person to be unable to feel or notice damage is occurring from a warm or cold application

2. Numbness, pain, blisters, or skin that is this color should be reported to the nurse

5. Type of application that increases blood flow to an injured area

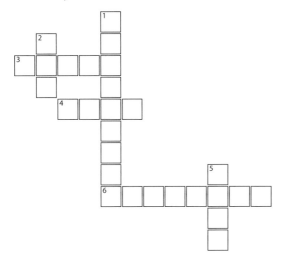

True or False

7. _____ Moisture reduces the effects of heat and cold.

8. _____ Dry applications are more likely to cause injury than moist applications.

9. _____ Redness, pain, blisters, and numbness are signs that an application may be causing tissue damage.

10. _____ A disposable warm pack is a type of dry application.

11. _____ Circulation to the perineal area is decreased when having a sitz bath.

12. _____ Sitz baths may stimulate voiding (urination).

13. _____ Residents may feel weak or dizzy after a sitz bath.

7. Discuss non-sterile and sterile dressings

Fill in the Blank

1. Sterile dressings cover new,

   _____,

   or _____
   wounds.

2. A _____
   changes sterile dressings.

3. Non-sterile dressings are applied to dry,

   _____
   wounds that have less chance of

   _____.

Short Answer

4. What may a nursing assistant be asked to do with regard to sterile dressings?

   _____

   _____

   _____

   _____

   _____

   _____

5. What are the supplies that may be needed for a sterile dressing change?

   _____

   _____

   _____

   _____

   _____

6. What should a nursing assistant observe and report about the wound site during sterile dressing changes?

   _____

   _____

   _____

   _____

   _____

8. Discuss guidelines for elastic bandages

Multiple Choice

1. Elastic bandages are also known as
   (A) Non-sterile bandages
   (B) Plastic bandages
   (C) Liquid bandages
   (D) Aseptic bandages

2. One purpose of elastic bandages is to
   (A) Elevate a cast
   (B) Hold a dressing in place
   (C) Cover pressure injuries
   (D) Help with ambulation

3. Elastic bandages should be applied snugly enough to control _____ and prevent movement of _____.
   (A) Temperature, the resident
   (B) Bleeding, dressings
   (C) Elevation, dressings
   (D) Movement, temperature

4. How soon should an NA check on a resident after applying a bandage?
   (A) 60 minutes
   (B) The next day
   (C) 2 hours
   (D) 10 minutes

9. List care guidelines for intravenous (IV) therapy

Multiple Choice

1. IV therapy allows direct access to
   (A) The joints
   (B) The lungs
   (C) The bloodstream
   (D) The muscles

2. What is the nursing assistant's responsibility for IV care?
   (A) Inserting IV lines
   (B) Removing IV lines
   (C) Care of the IV site
   (D) Documenting observations

3. If the fluid in an IV bag is nearly gone, the nursing assistant should
   (A) Add saline to the bag
   (B) Notify the nurse
   (C) Replace the bag with a new one
   (D) Reset the pump alarm

10. Discuss oxygen therapy and explain related care guidelines

Multiple Choice

1. Which of the following is a box-like device that changes air in the room into air with more oxygen?
   (A) Oxygen cannula
   (B) Oxygen face mask
   (C) Oxygen concentrator
   (D) Oxygen prongs

2. When should the nursing assistant administer a resident's oxygen?
   (A) Whenever the resident requests that she do so
   (B) According to the care plan
   (C) Once per shift
   (D) Never

3. What is the purpose of a nasal cannula?
   (A) To provide liquid nitrogen to the resident
   (B) To change the air in a room into air with more oxygen
   (C) To provide concentrated oxygen through a resident's nose
   (D) To secure a face mask to a resident who only occasionally needs oxygen

4. Liquid oxygen can cause which of the following?
   (A) Frostbite
   (B) Oxygen addiction
   (C) Digestive problems
   (D) Congestive heart failure

5. What kind of water is used in humidifying bottles for oxygen concentrators?
   (A) Sparkling water
   (B) Natural spring water
   (C) Distilled water
   (D) Tap water

6. What is the purpose of a humidifier?
   (A) To put only warm moisture in the air
   (B) To remove moisture from the air
   (C) To put warm or cool moisture in the air
   (D) To clean the air without adding moisture

15

Nutrition and Hydration

1. Describe the importance of proper nutrition and list the six basic nutrients

Short Answer

Write the letter of the correct basic nutrient beside each description below. Use W for water, C for carbohydrates, P for protein, F for fats, V for vitamins, and M for minerals.

1. _____ Sources include seafood, dried beans, poultry, and soy products.

2. _____ A person can only survive a few days without this.

3. _____ These build bones and help in blood formation.

4. _____ These add flavor to food and help to absorb certain vitamins.

5. _____ These are essential for tissue growth and repair.

6. _____ These may come from olives, nuts, and dairy products.

7. _____ The body cannot make most of these nutrients; they must be obtained through certain foods.

8. _____ These provide fiber, which is necessary for bowel elimination.

9. _____ Examples include bread, cereal, and potatoes.

10. _____ This is the most essential nutrient for life.

11. _____ Categories include monounsaturated and saturated.

12. _____ Through perspiration, this helps to maintain body temperature.

13. _____ Can be fat-soluble or water-soluble.

14. _____ These help the body store energy.

15. _____ Iron and calcium are examples.

2. Describe the USDA's MyPlate

Short Answer

The USDA developed the MyPlate icon and website to help promote healthy eating practices. Looking at the MyPlate icon, fill in the food groups.

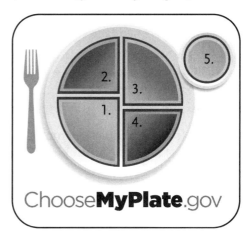

1. _____

2. _____

3. _____

4. _____

5. _____

6. Describe the last meal you ate. Organize the food into the MyPlate food groups and give an estimate of how much of each food group made up your plate.

_____

_____

_____

Nutrition and Hydration

_____
_____
_____
_____
_____
_____
_____
_____
_____
_____
_____
_____

Multiple Choice

7. MyPlate's guidelines state that half of a person's plate should be made up of
   (A) Grains and protein
   (B) Vegetables and fruits
   (C) Seafood and dairy
   (D) Grains and dairy

8. Out of the following choices, which color of vegetables has the best nutritional content?
   (A) Dark green
   (B) Pale yellow
   (C) Dark purple
   (D) Light brown

9. Most of a person's fruit choices should be
   (A) Fruit bars
   (B) Smoothies
   (C) Cut-up fruit
   (D) Fruit juice

10. What kinds of grains are best to consume?
    (A) Refined grains
    (B) White grains
    (C) Whole grains
    (D) Corn grains

11. Which of the following is considered a plant-based protein?
    (A) Salmon
    (B) Eggs
    (C) Sausage
    (D) Beans

12. Oatmeal and pasta are examples of foods made from which food group?
    (A) Vegetables
    (B) Fruits
    (C) Grains
    (D) Protein

13. Most dairy group choices should be
    (A) Whole-fat
    (B) 2% fat
    (C) Half and half
    (D) Low-fat

14. Which of the following foods is considered high in sodium?
    (A) Apple
    (B) Pickle
    (C) Avocado
    (D) Corn

3. Identify nutritional problems of the elderly or ill

Fill in the Blank

1. Encourage residents to
   _____.

2. Provide _____
   before and after meals.

3. Honor residents'
   _____ likes
   and dislikes.

4. Offer different kinds of foods and
   _____.

5. Allow enough _____
   to finish eating.

6. Notify the nurse if a resident has trouble using _____.

7. Position residents sitting
   _____ for eating.

8. If resident has had a loss of
   _____,
   ask about it.

9. Record meal/snack
   _____.

Short Answer

Make a check mark (✓) by all of the correct guidelines for working with residents who require tube feedings.

10. _____ The nursing assistant should remove the tube when the feeding is finished.

11. _____ During a feeding, the resident should remain in a sitting position with the head of the bed elevated at least 45 degrees.

12. _____ Redness or drainage around the opening should be reported.

13. _____ The nursing assistant is responsible for slowly pouring feedings into the tube.

14. _____ The nursing assistant should give careful skin care for residents who must remain in bed for long periods to help prevent pressure injuries.

15. _____ It is important for the nursing assistant to wash his hands before assisting in any way with a tube feeding.

16. _____ After a resident has had a tube feeding, the nursing assistant should help the resident lie down flat on his back.

4. Describe factors that influence food preferences

Short Answer

1. Briefly describe some of the foods you ate while growing up. Were there any special dishes your family made that were related to your culture, religion, or region?

_____

_____

_____

_____

_____

_____

_____

_____

_____

2. What rights do residents have with regard to food choices?

_____

_____

_____

_____

_____

_____

_____

5. Explain the role of the dietary department

Short Answer

1. What is the role of the dietary department?

_____

_____

_____

_____

_____

2. When planning meals, what does the dietary department consider?

_____

_____

_____

_____

_____

3. What information is contained on diet cards?

_____

_____

_____

_____

_____

6. Explain special diets

Matching
Read the following sentences and identify what special diet each is describing. Choose from the diets listed below. Use each letter only once.

1. _____ Bland Diet
2. _____ Diabetic Diet
3. _____ Fluid-Restricted Diet
4. _____ Gluten-Free Diet
5. _____ High-Potassium Diet
6. _____ High-Residue Diet
7. _____ Liquid Diet
8. _____ Low-Fat/Low-Cholesterol Diet
9. _____ Low-Protein Diet
10. _____ Low-Residue Diet
11. _____ Low-Sodium Diet
12. _____ Mechanical Soft Diet
13. _____ Modified Calorie Diet
14. _____ Pureed Diet
15. _____ Soft Diet
16. _____ Vegetarian Diet

(A) To prevent further heart or kidney damage, doctors may restrict fluid intake on this diet.

(B) This diet consists of foods that are in a liquid state at body temperature, and is usually ordered as clear or full.

(C) This diet consists of soft or chopped foods that are easy to chew; foods that are hard to chew and swallow, such as raw vegetables, will be restricted.

(D) People who have kidney disease may also be on this diet, which encourages foods like breads and pasta.

(E) People at risk for heart attacks and heart disease may be placed on this diet, which limits fatty and processed meats and fried foods.

(F) Carb counting may be part of this diet, as the amount of carbohydrates eaten must be carefully regulated.

(G) Salt is restricted in this diet.

(H) This diet is used for losing weight or preventing weight gain.

(I) The food used in this diet has been ground into a thick paste of baby-food consistency.

(J) Often used for people who have gastric ulcers, this diet involves avoiding alcohol, spicy foods, and citrus juices, among other items.

(K) Health reasons, a dislike of meat, a compassion for animals, or a belief in non-violence may lead a person to this diet.

(L) Used for people who have celiac disease, this diet eliminates foods containing wheat flour, such as tortillas, crackers, breads, and pasta.

(M) Foods high in this mineral will be encouraged in this diet; this includes bananas, prunes, dried apricots, figs, and sweet potatoes.

(N) This diet increases the amount of fiber and whole grains ingested; it helps prevent constipation.

(O) This diet is used for people with bowel disturbances and reduces the amount of fiber and whole grains ingested.

(P) Foods in this diet are chopped or blended and are prepared using blenders, food processors, or cutting utensils.

7. Explain thickened liquids and identify three basic thickened consistencies

True or False

1. _____ Thickening improves the ability to control fluids in the mouth and throat.

2. _____ A speech-language pathologist will evaluate the resident to determine the thickness that the resident requires.

3. _____ Beverages will always arrive pre-thickened from the dietary department.

4. _____ A resident who must have thickened liquids may drink regular water.

5. _____ Liquids that are nectar thick must be consumed with a spoon.

6. _____ A spoon should stand up straight in a glass of liquid that is pudding thick.

8. Describe how to make dining enjoyable for residents

Crossword

Across

1. Should be washed before residents eat

4. Proper position for eating that helps prevent swallowing problems

5. Something that has a positive effect on eating and helps prevent loneliness and boredom

Down

2. Use of eyeglasses, hearing aids, and these should be encouraged

3. Devices that can help residents with eating

6. Noise level should be kept _____ when residents are eating.

Scenarios

Read each scenario below and make suggestions for making mealtime more enjoyable for the resident.

7. Mrs. Peterson is a resident who is visually impaired. At mealtimes, she cannot see her food very well and complains that everything looks the same.

_____

_____

_____

_____

8. Mr. Leisering comes to dinner in his pajamas. His hair has not been brushed, and he is wearing slippers instead of shoes.

_____

_____

_____

_____

9. Ms. Lopez does not speak very much English, and she has not met any of the other Spanish-speaking residents. She comes to meals wrapped in a large sweater and jumps every time she hears trays clattering or when someone raises his voice.

_____

_____

_____

_____

_____

10. Mr. Gaines has dentures, but he says that they give him pain so he often does not wear them while eating. It takes him a long time to finish his meals, and he has to concentrate so hard on chewing his food that he does not seem interested in conversing with anyone around him.

_____

_____

_____

_____

9. Explain how to serve meal trays and assist with eating

True or False

1. _____ The nursing assistant should not rush a resident while he is eating.

2. _____ All residents sitting together at one table should be served at the same time so that they may eat together.

3. _____ It is important for the nursing assistant to identify each resident before serving a meal tray.

4. _____ The nursing assistant should remain standing while feeding a resident.

Name: _____

5. ____ If a resident needs his food cut up, it should be done before the food is brought to the table.

6. ____ The resident's mouth should be empty before the nursing assistant offers another bite of food.

7. ____ Using a straw is helpful for a resident who has a swallowing problem.

8. ____ Pureed food should not be seasoned.

9. ____ To promote a healthy appetite, the nursing assistant should remain silent while helping a resident eat.

10. ____ If food is too hot, the nursing assistant should blow on it for a few minutes until it is cool enough for the resident to eat.

11. ____ Residents should be sitting upright at a 90-degree angle for eating.

12. ____ If a resident wants to eat his dessert first, the nursing assistant should explain that it is unhealthy and that he should begin with his entree.

13. ____ Alternating cold and hot foods or bland foods and sweets can help increase appetite.

14. ____ The nursing assistant should refer to pureed carrots as "orange stuff" so the resident knows which food the NA is talking about.

Scenarios

Read each scenario below and describe how each NA can improve her technique of assisting at meals.

15. Mrs. Rains, a Catholic resident, asks Carol to join her in a small prayer before she eats. Carol declines, explaining that she does not believe in God and thinks that prayer is pointless.

_____

_____

_____

_____

_____

16. Tracy had a fight with her husband this morning and is in a very bad mood. Mrs. Foster, a friendly resident, tries to make conversation as Tracy is handing out meal trays. "I don't have time to talk right now," Tracy snaps at her. "Can't you see how much I have to do?"

_____

_____

_____

_____

_____

_____

17. Mr. Parks, a resident with arthritis, can usually feed himself, but today his hands are hurting him so much that he cannot hold the utensils or even his napkin. Carol helps him eat while joking loudly with the other residents that he must be feeling like royalty having someone wait on him hand and foot.

_____

_____

_____

_____

_____

18. Mr. Correll is recovering from pneumonia. Pam serves his meal and then watches for a few moments to see if he needs any help. When she determines that he can feed himself, she goes on to help another resident. After she leaves, Mr. Correll starts to feel weak and begins having trouble lifting the utensils to his mouth. He waits 15 minutes for someone to come back to help him finish his meal.

_____

_____

_____

_____

19. While handing out meal trays, Pam notices that Mr. Gray's diet card indicates a low-sodium diet but his meal tray contains a meal for residents with no restrictions. She assumes his diet must have changed and gives him the tray.

_____

_____

_____

_____

_____

_____

20. Mrs. Palmer has Parkinson's disease. She can feed herself, but she does so very slowly, as her hands are sometimes shaky. Tracy cuts Mrs. Palmer's food and feeds it to her so that it will not take her so long to finish.

_____

_____

_____

_____

_____

_____

_____

10. Describe how to assist residents with special needs

Fill in the Blank

1. Use _____ devices such as utensils with built-up handle grips, plate guards, and drinking cups when necessary.

2. For a resident who is visually impaired, use the face of an imaginary

_____

to explain the position of what is in front of her.

3. For a resident who has had a stroke, place food in the unaffected, or

_____,

side of the mouth.

4. A resident with Parkinson's disease may need help if

_____

or shaking make it difficult for them to eat.

5. The hand-over-hand approach is an example of a physical

_____

that can help promote independence.

6. Verbal cues must be short and

_____

and prompt the resident to do something.

7. If a resident has poor sitting balance, seat him in a regular dining room chair with armrests, rather than in a

_____.

Put the resident in the proper position in the chair, which means hips are at a

_____ -

degree angle, knees are flexed, and feet and arms are fully supported.

8. If a resident bites down on utensils, ask him to

_____

his mouth.

9. If a resident pockets food in his cheeks, ask him to chew and

_____

the food.

11. Define *dysphagia* and identify signs and symptoms of swallowing problems

Multiple Choice

1. The medical term for difficulty swallowing is
   (A) Aspiration
   (B) Dysphagia
   (C) Edema
   (D) Cyanosis

2. In order to prevent aspiration, the nursing assistant should keep the resident in the _____ position after eating for at least 30 minutes.
    (A) Upright
    (B) Lying flat
    (C) Reclining
    (D) Side

3. Food should always be placed in the _____ side of the mouth.
    (A) Top
    (B) Weaker
    (C) Left
    (D) Stronger

12. Explain intake and output (I&O)

True or False

1. _____ Fluids come in the form of liquids that a person drinks, as well as semi-liquid foods such as soup or gelatin.

2. _____ The fluid a person consumes is called intake or input.

3. _____ All of the body's fluid output is in the form of urine.

4. _____ Fluid balance is taking in and eliminating the same amounts of fluid.

5. _____ Most people need to consciously monitor their fluid balance.

Conversions

6. A healthy person generally needs to take in about 64 ounces (oz) of fluid each day. How many milliliters (mL) is this?

    _____

    How many cups is this?

    _____

7. Mrs. Hedman drinks half a glass of orange juice. The glass holds about 1 cup of liquid. How many milliliters of orange juice did Mrs. Hedman drink?

    _____

8. Mr. Ramirez just ate some chocolate pudding from a 6-ounce container. The leftover pudding measures about 35 milliliters (mL). How many milliliters of pudding did Mr. Ramirez eat?

    _____

9. Miss Sumiko has a bowl of soup for lunch. The soup bowl holds about 1½ cups of liquid. How many milliliters is this?

    _____

    Miss Sumiko finishes most of her soup, but there are about 25 milliliters left. How many milliliters of soup did Miss Sumiko eat?

    _____

10. After his lunch, Mr. Lake selects orange gelatin for dessert. He is given one cup of gelatin, but he only eats about ¼ of it. How many milliliters (mL) of gelatin did he consume?

    _____

    _____

    How many milliliters were left over?

    _____

11. Mr. Weiss indicates that he needs to use the bathroom. He uses a urinal to help with measurement of his output. According to the container, Mr. Lake urinated two cups of urine. How many milliliters (mL) is this?

    _____

Multiple Choice

12. A resident drinks six ounces of water. How many milliliters is this?
    (A) 120 mL
    (B) 160 mL
    (C) 180 mL
    (D) 200 mL

13. How many ounces are equal to 30 milliliters?
    (A) 1 ounce
    (B) 10 ounces
    (C) 15 ounces
    (D) 30 ounces

14. A resident's urine measures ¾ cup in a graduate. How many ounces is this?
    (A) 4 ounces
    (B) 6 ounces
    (C) 8 ounces
    (D) 10 ounces

15. A 12-ounce container of fluid is equal to how many milliliters (mL)?
    (A) 360 mL
    (B) 280 mL
    (C) 120 mL
    (D) 240 mL

Labeling

List the amount of fluid in milliliters (mL) in each container.

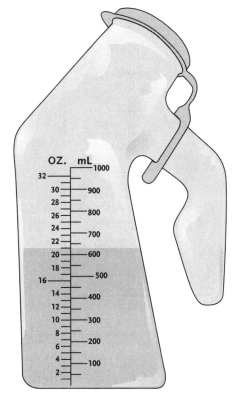

17. _____

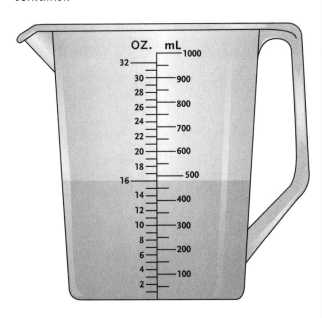

16. _____

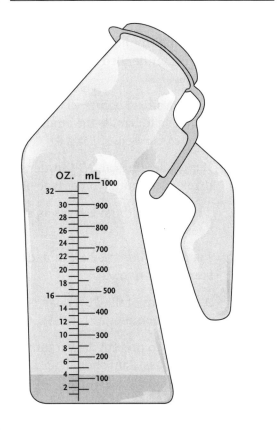

18. _____

Name: _____

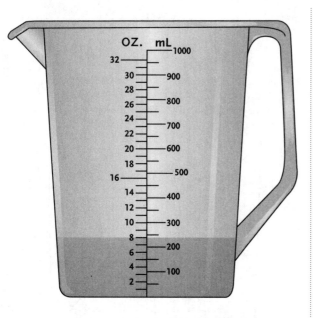

19. _____

10. _____ The NA should make sure that the water pitcher and cup are light enough for the resident to lift.

13. Identify ways to assist residents in maintaining fluid balance

True or False

1. _____ Twenty-six ounces of water per day is the recommended amount for most people.

2. _____ Fluid overload occurs when the body is unable to handle the amount of fluid consumed.

3. _____ If a resident has an NPO order, he can drink water but no other type of fluid.

4. _____ The sense of thirst lessens as a person ages.

5. _____ People can become dehydrated by vomiting too much.

6. _____ A symptom of fluid overload is edema of the extremities.

7. _____ In order to prevent dehydration, the nursing assistant should offer fresh fluids to residents often.

8. _____ One symptom of dehydration is dark urine.

9. _____ A resident who has a swallowing problem should suck on ice chips regularly.

16

Urinary Elimination

1. List qualities of urine and identify signs and symptoms about urine to report

Multiple Choice

1. Urine is made up of water and
   (A) Dye
   (B) Blood
   (C) Waste products
   (D) Plasma

2. Adults usually produce approximately _____ milliliters (mL) of urine per day.
   (A) 2400 to 2800
   (B) 25 to 50
   (C) 400 to 700
   (D) 1200 to 1500

3. How should urine normally appear?
   (A) Pale yellow
   (B) Rust-colored
   (C) Red
   (D) Cloudy

4. Another word for urinating is
   (A) Expiring
   (B) Circulating
   (C) Voiding
   (D) Digesting

Short Answer

Mark an X next to each of the following items that is a sign or symptom that should be reported to the nurse.

5. _____ Urinary incontinence

6. _____ Urine has faint smell

7. _____ Urine is pale yellow in color

8. _____ Blood in urine

9. _____ Urine is transparent

10. _____ Painful urination

11. _____ Glucose in urine

12. _____ Cloudy urine

13. _____ Urine has a fruity smell

14. _____ Dark urine

15. _____ Urine has a strong smell

2. List factors affecting urination and demonstrate how to assist with elimination

True or False

1. _____ As a person ages, the bladder is not able to hold the same amount of urine as it once did.

2. _____ Diuretics are medications that can cause frequent urination.

3. _____ When assisting with perineal care, the nursing assistant should wipe from back to front.

4. _____ A healthy person needs at least 64 ounces of fluid each day.

5. _____ Closing the bathroom door is a way to promote a resident's privacy while she is urinating.

6. _____ The sense of thirst increases as a person ages, causing him to be thirsty more often.

7. _____ Caffeine can increase urine output.

8. _____ Diabetes can affect urination.

Name: _____

Multiple Choice

9. A fracture pan is used for urination for
   (A) Any resident who cannot get out of bed
   (B) Residents who cannot raise their hips
   (C) Residents who have problems with urinary incontinence
   (D) Residents who have difficulty urinating

10. Men will generally use a _____ for urination when they cannot get out of bed.
    (A) Urinal
    (B) Fracture pan
    (C) Toilet
    (D) Portable commode

11. Residents who can get out of bed but cannot walk to the bathroom may use a(n)
    (A) Toilet
    (B) Urinal
    (C) Portable commode
    (D) Indwelling catheter

12. Another name for portable commode is
    (A) Toilet attachment
    (B) Portable urinal
    (C) Bedside commode
    (D) Hat

13. Which of the following statements is true?
    (A) When handling body wastes, the nursing assistant should wear gloves.
    (B) The nursing assistant should put the waste container on the overbed table.
    (C) The nursing assistant should store elimination equipment on the resident's side table.
    (D) Containers used for elimination should be cleaned after every two uses.

3. Describe common diseases and disorders of the urinary system

True or False

1. _____ Urinary tract infections are more common in men than in women.

2. _____ Urine irritates the skin and must be completely cleaned off.

3. _____ Functional incontinence is caused by overflow of the bladder.

4. _____ Kidney stones form when urine crystallizes in the kidneys.

5. _____ Kidney dialysis is used for cleaning mucus from the lungs.

6. _____ When a person has a urinary tract infection, she may experience a painful burning sensation during urination.

7. _____ To avoid infection, women should wipe the perineal area from front to back after elimination.

8. _____ Kidney stones can be the result of a lack of fluid intake.

9. _____ Excessive salt in the diet can cause damage to the kidneys.

10. _____ Urinary incontinence is a normal part of getting older.

11. _____ Urinary incontinence can occur if a resident is bedbound, ill, elderly, paralyzed, or injured.

12. _____ Stress incontinence is involuntary voiding due to an abrupt urge.

13. _____ It is disrespectful for a nursing assistant to refer to incontinence briefs as *diapers*.

4. Describe guidelines for urinary catheter care

Matching
Use each letter only once.

1. _____ Catheter

2. _____ Condom catheter

3. _____ Indwelling catheter

4. _____ Straight catheter

5. _____ Urinary catheter

(A) Urinary catheter that has an attachment that fits onto the penis

(B) Urinary catheter that is removed immediately after urine is drained

(C) Thin tube used to drain urine from the bladder

(D) Urinary catheter that stays inside the bladder for a period of time

(E) Thin tube inserted into the body that is used to drain or inject fluids

Short Answer

6. List three guidelines to follow when working around residents with catheters.

_____

_____

_____

_____

_____

_____

_____

_____

7. List six things to report to the nurse about a resident's catheter.

_____

_____

_____

_____

_____

_____

_____

_____

5. Identify types of urine specimens that are collected

Matching
Use each letter only once.

1. ____   24-hour urine specimen

2. ____   Clean-catch specimen

3. ____   Hat

4. ____   Routine urine specimen

5. ____   Specimen

(A) Collection container sometimes put into the toilet bowl to collect samples

(B) Urine sample collected any time a resident voids

(C) Also called *mid-stream* specimen

(D) A sample that is used for analysis in order to try to make a diagnosis

(E) Collects all urine voided in 24 hours

6. Explain types of tests performed on urine

Multiple Choice

1. A reagent strip
    (A) Tests for food in urine
    (B) Tests for pH level in urine
    (C) Tests for illegal drugs in urine
    (D) Tests for fat in urine

2. The presence of glucose or ketones in urine may be a sign of
    (A) High blood pressure
    (B) Thyroid disorder
    (C) Anemia
    (D) Diabetes

3. Occult blood in urine is
    (A) A normal change of aging
    (B) Easily seen
    (C) Hidden
    (D) A sign of anemia

Name: _____

4. A urine specific gravity test
   (A) Checks for adequate oxygen levels
   (B) Indicates the specific type of urinary incontinence
   (C) Counts amount of blood cells in urine
   (D) Shows how density of urine compares to water

5. A double-voided urine specimen may be used to test for
   (A) Glucose
   (B) Sweat
   (C) Sputum
   (D) Nitrite

7. Explain guidelines for assisting with bladder retraining

Scenarios

Ms. Potter has been staying at the Cool River Retirement Center for several months while she recovers from a broken hip. Her recovery is proceeding well, but she has had a problem with urinary incontinence since her injury. Her doctor tells the nurses and nursing assistants (NAs) on Ms. Potter's unit to assist her with bladder retraining. Below are examples of how three of the NAs help Ms. Potter with retraining. Read each one and state what the NA is doing well and/or what he or she should do differently.

1. Hannah, a new NA, wants to be very professional about the episodes of incontinence. While she is cleaning the bed, she remains very upbeat and friendly and does not mention the incontinence unless Ms. Potter brings it up.

   _____
   _____
   _____
   _____
   _____
   _____
   _____
   _____

2. Greta senses Ms. Potter's acute embarrassment and it makes her nervous. Whenever she has to assist Ms. Potter with retraining efforts, she speaks very little and does not make eye contact with her. She tries to finish her work as quickly as possible to limit Ms. Potter's discomfort.

   _____
   _____
   _____
   _____
   _____
   _____
   _____
   _____

3. Pete has been very encouraging and positive with Ms. Potter. He has charted her bathroom schedule. He makes sure to be available to help her around the usual times that she needs to go to the bathroom. He responds to her call light quickly.

   _____
   _____
   _____
   _____
   _____
   _____
   _____
   _____
   _____

17

Bowel Elimination

1. List qualities of stool and identify signs and symptoms about stool to report

True or False

1. _____ Defecation is the process of passing feces from the large intestine out of the body.

2. _____ Everyone should have the same number of bowel movements per day.

3. _____ Normal stool is watery and loose.

4. _____ Certain foods can change the color of stool.

5. _____ Stool that is whitish, black, or red should be reported to the nurse.

6. _____ Constipation is normal and does not need to be reported to the nurse.

7. _____ Fecal incontinence is normal for people over age 65.

2. List factors affecting bowel elimination

Multiple Choice

1. Peristalsis is
   (A) Decreased saliva production that occurs as a person ages
   (B) Contractions that move food through the gastrointestinal system
   (C) Pain that can occur during elimination
   (D) The involuntary loss of stool

2. Foods that are high in animal fats and refined sugars but low in fiber can
   (A) Improve bowel elimination
   (B) Cause constipation
   (C) Cause gluten intolerance
   (D) Cause weight loss

3. Normal bowel elimination is aided by
   (A) Proper fluid intake
   (B) Eating mostly red meat
   (C) Eating dairy products, such as cheese
   (D) All-liquid diets

4. The best position for bowel elimination is
   (A) Lying supine on the back
   (B) Lying prone on the abdomen
   (C) Reclining 45 degrees
   (D) Squatting and leaning forward

5. Bowel elimination usually occurs
   (A) Morning, midday, and night
   (B) After meals
   (C) In the supine position
   (D) During physical activity

3. Describe common diseases and disorders of the gastrointestinal system

Crossword

Across

6. The frequent elimination of liquid or semi-liquid feces

8. Enlarged veins in the rectum that cause itching and burning

Down

1. Residents with peptic ulcers should avoid drinks containing this ingredient, as well as beverages containing alcohol

2. May result from untreated heartburn

3. The diversion of waste to an artificial opening (stoma) through the abdomen

Name: _____

4. Keeping the body in this position during sleep may help symptoms of gastroesophageal reflux disease

5. Treatment of constipation often includes increasing the amount of this eaten

7. Abbreviation for gastroesophageal reflux disease

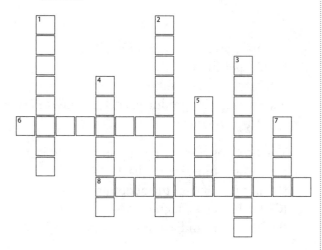

4. Discuss how enemas are given

Short Answer

1. Why are enemas given?

_____

_____

_____

_____

_____

_____

2. What position must a resident be in when getting an enema?

_____

_____

_____

3. If the resident has pain or if the nursing assistant feels resistance while giving an enema, what should the NA do?

_____

_____

_____

_____

4. How can the resident's legal rights be protected while giving an enema?

_____

_____

_____

_____

_____

_____

_____

5. Demonstrate how to collect a stool specimen

True or False

1. _____ Stool is often tested for blood, pathogens, or worms.

2. _____ An ova and parasites test is used to detect occult blood in stool.

3. _____ Ova and parasites tests must be done while the stool is still warm.

4. _____ Urine or toilet paper can ruin a stool sample.

6. Explain occult blood testing

Fill in the Blank

1. Hidden blood in stool is called

_____

blood.

2. Blood in stool may be a sign of a serious problem, such as

_____

or other illnesses.

7. Define *ostomy* and list care guidelines

True or False

1. _____ An ostomy is the surgical creation of an opening from an area inside the body to the outside.

2. ____ The artificial opening in the abdomen through which stool is eliminated is called a stoma.

3. ____ Residents who have ileostomies will need to restrict their fluid intake.

4. ____ The nursing assistant should wear gloves when providing ostomy care.

Short Answer

5. Why might a resident be embarrassed by his ostomy?

   _____

   _____

   _____

   _____

Multiple Choice

6. How often should an ostomy bag be emptied and cleaned or replaced?
   (A) Once a day
   (B) Every hour
   (C) Whenever a stool is eliminated
   (D) Before a resident gets out of bed for the day

7. What could cause a food blockage in a resident who has an ileostomy?
   (A) Too much liquid in the resident's diet
   (B) A large amount of high-fiber food in the resident's diet
   (C) Skin irritation
   (D) Cold compresses

8. Explain guidelines for assisting with bowel retraining

Fill in the Blank

1. Residents who have had a disruption in their bowel _____
   may need help to restore normal
   _____.

2. Wear _____
   when handling body wastes.

3. Explain the training
   _____ to the resident.
   Keep a _____ of
   the resident's bowel habits.

4. Encourage plenty of
   _____
   and foods that are high in
   _____.

5. Provide _____
   for elimination in the bed and bathroom.

6. Help with _____
   care, which can prevent skin breakdown.

7. Discard clothing _____
   and _____
   briefs properly.

8. Praise _____
   or _____
   to control bowels.

9. Never show _____
   or _____
   toward a resident who is incontinent.

Bowel Elimination

18

Common Chronic and Acute Conditions

1. Describe common diseases and disorders of the integumentary system

Matching
Use each letter only once.

1. ____ Dermatitis

2. ____ Fungal infection

3. ____ Scabies

4. ____ Shingles

5. ____ Wound

(A) Caused by fungal imbalances; athlete's foot, vaginal yeast infections, and *tinea* are examples

(B) Contagious skin condition caused by a tiny mite that burrows into the skin, where it lays eggs, causing intense itching and a skin rash

(C) A type of injury to the skin; classified as either open or closed

(D) Skin rash caused by the varicella-zoster virus (VZV), which is the same virus that causes chickenpox

(E) A general term that refers to an inflammation, or swelling, of the skin

2. Describe common diseases and disorders of the musculoskeletal system

Multiple Choice

Arthritis

1. Arthritis is a general term referring to _____ of the joints.
   (A) Immobility
   (B) Swelling
   (C) Redness
   (D) Stiffness

2. Arthritis may be the result of
   (A) Congestive heart failure
   (B) Amputation
   (C) Autoimmune illness
   (D) Substance abuse

3. What happens to the body when a person suffers from an autoimmune illness?
   (A) The circulatory system stops functioning, and blood backs up into the heart.
   (B) The immune system attacks diseased tissue in the body.
   (C) The immune system attacks normal tissue in the body.
   (D) The musculoskeletal system becomes diseased.

4. Osteoarthritis is common in
   (A) The elderly
   (B) Infants
   (C) Teenagers
   (D) Nursing assistants

5. The pain and stiffness of osteoarthritis may increase with
   (A) Hot weather
   (B) Cold weather
   (C) An active lifestyle
   (D) Dehydration

6. Rheumatoid arthritis affects the _____ joints first.
   (A) Smaller
   (B) Larger
   (C) Elbow
   (D) There is no typical progression.

7. Arthritis is generally treated with
   (A) Surgical removal of the affected limb
   (B) Application of a cast to immobilize the affected area
   (C) Deep breathing exercises
   (D) Anti-inflammatory medications

Osteoporosis

True or False

8. _____ Osteoporosis causes bones to become brittle and break easily.

9. _____ Residents with osteoporosis must be moved very carefully.

10. _____ Osteoporosis is more common in women before menopause.

11. _____ A lack of regular exercise is one cause of osteoporosis.

12. _____ Osteoporosis cannot be treated.

Fractures

Multiple Choice

13. When caring for a resident who has a cast, the NA should _____ the extremity that is in a cast to stop swelling.
    (A) Lower
    (B) Double bandage
    (C) Elevate
    (D) Shake

14. The cast should be kept _____ and clean at all times.
    (A) Dry
    (B) Wet
    (C) Hot
    (D) Flexed

15. A bone must be unable to _____ to allow the fusion of fractured parts.
    (A) Align
    (B) Heal
    (C) Strengthen
    (D) Move

16. Signs and symptoms of a fracture include
    (A) Moistness at the site
    (B) Coldness at the site
    (C) Swelling at the site
    (D) Dryness at the site

17. Fractures are broken bones and are often caused by
    (A) A high-fat diet
    (B) Hypertension
    (C) Osteoporosis
    (D) Dermatitis

18. When can a resident insert something inside the cast?
    (A) When skin itches
    (B) After the cast dries
    (C) When the cast is wet
    (D) Never

19. A fracture that has penetrated the skin and carries a high risk of infection is called a(n)
    (A) Open fracture
    (B) Hairline fracture
    (C) Closed fracture
    (D) Infectious fracture

20. Casts are generally made of
    (A) Metal
    (B) Fiberglass
    (C) Wool
    (D) Rubber

Hip Fractures

True or False

21. _____ Most fractured hips require surgery.

22. _____ The nursing assistant should perform range of motion exercises on the operative leg to help with healing.

23. _____ Preventing falls is an important part of preventing hip fractures.

24. _____ Elderly people heal slowly and are at risk for secondary illnesses.

25. _____ The nursing assistant may disconnect the traction assembly if the resident requests it.

26. _____ When transferring a resident from the bed, a pillow should be used between the thighs to keep the legs separated.

27. _____ The NA should begin with the unaffected, or stronger, side first when dressing a resident who is recovering from a hip replacement.

28. _____ The stronger side always leads in standing, pivoting, and sitting.

Multiple Choice

29. What is the main reason that hip fractures are more common in the elderly?
    (A) Bones weaken as people age.
    (B) Elderly people get too much exercise.
    (C) Elderly people are depressed.
    (D) Elderly people can bear more weight on their bones.

30. Which side of the body should a resident recovering from a hip replacement dress first?
    (A) Affected/weaker side
    (B) Right side
    (C) Unaffected/stronger side
    (D) Left side

31. What does the abbreviation *PWB* stand for?
    (A) Previously weakened bones
    (B) Partial weight-bearing
    (C) Patient's weight before
    (D) Patient wants baths

32. If a nursing assistant sees *NWB* on a resident's care plan, the resident
    (A) Can support 100 percent of his body weight on one leg
    (B) Can support some weight, but not all, on one or both legs
    (C) Is unable to support any weight on one or both legs
    (D) Can use stairs without assistance

Knee Replacement

True or False

33. _____ A knee replacement may be done to relieve pain or restore motion to the knee.

34. _____ The recovery time for a knee replacement is longer than for a hip replacement.

35. _____ Compression stockings are applied to the legs and hooked to a machine that inflates and deflates to act as the muscles normally would.

36. _____ Ankle pumps are simple exercises to promote circulation to the legs.

37. _____ Fluid intake should be restricted after a knee replacement.

Muscular Dystrophy (MD)

True or False

38. _____ Muscular dystrophy (MD) is an inherited disease that causes gradual wasting away of the muscles.

39. _____ Most forms of MD become apparent in middle adulthood.

40. _____ Many forms of MD are very slow to progress.

41. _____ In the late stages of MD, the nursing assistant may need to perform activities of daily living (ADLs) for the resident.

Amputation

Short Answer

42. What is phantom limb pain? Is it real?

    _____

    _____

    _____

    _____

    _____

3. Describe common diseases and disorders of the nervous system

CVA or Stroke

True or False

1. _____ A resident who has paralysis after a stroke will usually not require physical therapy.

2. _____ Range of motion exercises strengthen muscles and keep joints mobile.

3. _____ Leg exercises help improve circulation.

4. _____ When helping with transfers or ambulation, the nursing assistant should stand on the resident's stronger side.

5. _____ The NA should always use a gait belt for safety when helping a resident who has had a stroke to walk.

6. ____ The NA should refer to the side that has been affected by stroke as the bad side so that the resident will understand which side the NA is talking about.

7. ____ Gestures and smiles are important when communicating with a resident who has had a stroke.

8. ____ A resident who suffers confusion or memory loss due to a stroke may feel more secure if the NA establishes a routine of care.

9. ____ A resident who has a loss of sensation could easily burn himself.

10. ____ Food should always be placed in the unaffected, or stronger, side of the mouth.

11. ____ When assisting with dressing a resident who has had a stroke, the NA should dress the stronger side first.

Scenarios

Read each of the following statements and answer the questions.

12. Jody, a nursing assistant, is getting ready to help feed Mr. Elliot, who is recovering from a stroke. Mr. Elliot has difficulty communicating and also suffers from confusion. "Let's see," Jody says, "for lunch you have soup, a sandwich, and a salad. Now, what would you like to eat?" What is wrong with the way Jody is communicating with Mr. Elliot?

_____

_____

_____

_____

_____

_____

_____

13. Mr. Elliot's daughter visits during mealtime and asks how her dad is doing. Jody says, "Mr. Elliot is having trouble today with his eating. Just look at him. He's spilled water all

over himself." What is wrong with what Jody has just said?

_____

_____

_____

_____

_____

_____

_____

14. Jody notices that Mr. Elliot seems to be having trouble saying words clearly. He is beginning to get frustrated because he cannot tell Jody what he wants. Jody decides to ask only yes or no questions, so she tells Mr. Elliot, "If you find it too difficult to speak right now, why don't you try nodding your head for yes and shaking your head for no." What is Jody doing right?

_____

_____

_____

_____

_____

_____

_____

_____

Parkinson's Disease

True or False

15. ____ Parkinson's disease is a progressive disease that causes a section of the brain to degenerate.

16. ____ Parkinson's disease causes a shuffling gait and a mask-like facial expression.

17. ____ Pill-rolling is something that people with Parkinson's disease must do before taking their medication.

18. _____ A resident with Parkinson's disease should be discouraged from performing her own care to help save energy.

Multiple Sclerosis (MS)

Fill in the Blank

19. Multiple sclerosis causes the protective

_____

for the nerves, spinal cord, and white matter of the brain to break down over time.

20. For a person with MS, nerves cannot send

_____

to and from the brain in a normal way.

21. Symptoms of MS include

_____

vision, fatigue, tremors, poor balance, and difficulty walking.

22. The nursing assistant (NA) should offer _____ periods as necessary for residents with MS.

23. The NA should give residents plenty of time to _____ because people with MS often have trouble forming their thoughts.

24. _____ can worsen the effects of MS, so the NA should remain calm and listen to residents when they want to talk.

Head and Spinal Cord Injuries

True or False

25. _____ The effects of a spinal cord injury depend on the location of the injury and the force of impact.

26. _____ The lower the injury on the spinal cord, the greater the loss of function will be.

27. _____ Quadriplegia is a loss of function of the lower body and legs.

28. _____ Rehabilitation is of little help for people who have had spinal cord injuries.

29. _____ A resident with a head or spinal cord injury will need emotional support as well as physical help.

30. _____ A resident with a spinal cord injury may not feel a burn because of a loss of sensation.

31. _____ The NA should help the resident change positions at least every two hours to prevent pressure injuries.

32. _____ A resident with a spinal cord injury should drink very little fluid to prevent urinary tract infections.

Epilepsy

Short Answer

33. What causes epilepsy and how is epilepsy often treated?

_____

_____

_____

_____

_____

_____

_____

_____

_____

_____

Vision Impairment

Multiple Choice

34. What happens when a cataract develops?
    (A) The lens of the eye slowly disappears.
    (B) The lens of the eye becomes cloudy.
    (C) The lens of the eye stops functioning.
    (D) The lens of the eye becomes swollen.

35. How is glaucoma often treated?
    (A) With eye drops
    (B) By surgical removal of the optic nerve
    (C) With special eyeglasses
    (D) By reducing the amount of light in the room or area

36. How is diabetic retinopathy treated?
    (A) With laser treatment
    (B) By retinal transplant
    (C) With weight loss
    (D) With cool ice packs

Name: _____

4. Describe common diseases and disorders of the circulatory system

Hypertension (HTN) or High Blood Pressure

Short Answer

1. What is the consistent blood pressure measurement at which a person is diagnosed as having hypertension?

_____

_____

_____

2. What are three possible causes of hypertension?

_____

_____

_____

_____

_____

3. Why is treatment of hypertension important?

_____

_____

_____

_____

_____

Coronary Artery Disease (CAD)

True or False

4. _____ Coronary artery disease (CAD) occurs when the coronary arteries widen and increase blood flow.

5. _____ CAD lowers the supply of blood, oxygen, and nutrients to the heart and can lead to heart attack or stroke.

6. _____ Angina pectoris is chest pain, pressure, or discomfort caused by reduced oxygen to the heart.

7. _____ The heart needs more oxygen when the body is at rest.

8. _____ The pain of angina pectoris is usually described as pressure or tightness in the left side of the chest.

9. _____ A person suffering from angina pectoris may sweat, look pale, and have trouble breathing.

10. _____ If a person with CAD rests, it helps the blood flow return to normal.

11. _____ The nursing assistants can administer nitroglycerin to the resident if requested.

12. _____ A resident with CAD may need to avoid heavy meals and intense exercise.

Myocardial Infarction (MI) or Heart Attack

Short Answer

13. What causes a myocardial infarction (MI)?

_____

_____

_____

_____

_____

_____

_____

Congestive Heart Failure (CHF)

Fill in the Blank

14. Congestive heart failure can be treated and controlled with

_____.

15. Medications help remove excess

_____.

This means more trips to the

_____.

16. Limited _____
or _____
may be prescribed.

17. Residents may need to be

_____

at the same time every day.

18. Extra _____
may help residents who have trouble
breathing.

19. A common side effect of CHF medication is
_____.

Peripheral Vascular Disease (PVD)

Multiple Choice

20. Peripheral vascular disease (PVD) is a condi-
tion in which the legs, feet, arms, or hands
do not have enough
(A) Flexibility
(B) Fat
(C) Blood circulation
(D) Fluids

21. PVD is caused by
(A) Weakened bones
(B) Weakened heart muscle due to damage
(C) Infection of the lymph nodes
(D) Fatty deposits in blood vessels

22. When should anti-embolic hose be applied?
(A) Before the resident gets out of bed
(B) While the resident is walking around
(C) Right after a shower or tub bath
(D) During meal time

5. Describe common diseases and disorders of the respiratory system

Chronic Obstructive Pulmonary Disease (COPD)

Multiple Choice

1. Residents with chronic obstructive pulmo-
nary disease (COPD) have difficulty with
(A) Breathing
(B) Urination
(C) Losing weight
(D) Vision

2. For a person with COPD, a common fear is
(A) Constipation
(B) Incontinence
(C) Not being able to breathe
(D) Heart attack

3. The best position for a resident with
COPD is
(A) Lying flat on his back
(B) Sitting upright
(C) Lying on his stomach
(D) Lying on his side

4. Part of the nursing assistant's role in caring
for a resident with COPD includes
(A) Being calm and supportive
(B) Adjusting oxygen levels
(C) Making changes in the resident's diet
(D) Doing everything for the resident as
much as possible

5. Chronic bronchitis and emphysema are
grouped under
(A) Chronic obstructive pulmonary disease,
or COPD
(B) Muscular dystrophy, or MD
(C) Hypertension, or HTN
(D) Coronary artery disease, or CAD

Matching
Use each letter only once.

6. _____ Asthma

7. _____ Bronchiectasis

8. _____ Lung cancer

9. _____ Tuberculosis (TB)

10. _____ Upper respiratory infection (URI)

(A) Highly contagious lung disease; symptoms
include coughing, low-grade fever, shortness
of breath, weight loss, and fatigue

(B) Results from a viral infection of the nose,
sinuses, and throat; commonly called a cold

(C) Chronic inflammatory disease that occurs
when the respiratory system reacts strongly
to irritants, infection, cold air, or to allergens;
causes coughing and difficulty breathing

(D) Growth of abnormal cells or tumors in the
lungs

(E) Condition in which the bronchial tubes are
abnormally enlarged; causes chronic
coughing

6. Describe common diseases and disorders of the endocrine system

Diabetes

Multiple Choice

1. Diabetes is a condition in which the pancreas does not produce enough or does not properly use
   (A) Insulin
   (B) Glucose
   (C) Growth hormones
   (D) Adrenaline

2. Sugars collecting in the blood cause problems with
   (A) Breathing
   (B) Circulation
   (C) Pain level
   (D) Ambulation

3. Type 1 diabetes
   (A) Continues throughout a person's life
   (B) Is most common in the elderly
   (C) Is first treated with surgery
   (D) Does not require a change of diet

4. Changes in the circulatory system from diabetes can cause
   (A) Hair loss
   (B) Heart attack and stroke
   (C) Multiple sclerosis
   (D) COPD

5. The most common form of diabetes is
   (A) Pre-diabetes
   (B) Gestational diabetes
   (C) Type 1 diabetes
   (D) Type 2 diabetes

6. Poor circulation and impaired wound healing may result in
   (A) Urinary tract infections
   (B) Cancer
   (C) Leg and foot ulcers
   (D) An autoimmune disease

7. Gangrene can lead to
   (A) Loss of bowel control
   (B) Peripheral vascular disease
   (C) Congestive heart failure
   (D) Amputation

8. What condition occurs when a person's blood glucose level is above normal but not high enough for a diagnosis of type 2 diabetes?
   (A) Gestational diabetes
   (B) Type 1 diabetes
   (C) Pre-diabetes
   (D) Hyperglycemia

9. Careful _____ care is vitally important for people with diabetes.
   (A) Foot
   (B) Hair
   (C) Facial
   (D) Mouth

10. For a resident who has diabetes, where should lotion not be applied?
    (A) Upper arms
    (B) Lower back
    (C) Back of the legs
    (D) Between the toes

Hyperthyroidism and Hypothyroidism

Short Answer

11. What is hyperthyroidism?

_____

_____

_____

_____

_____

12. What is hypothyroidism?

_____

_____

_____

_____

7. Describe common diseases and disorders of the reproductive system

True or False

1. _____ Gonorrhea is easier to detect in men than in women.

2. ____ Genital herpes can be cured with antibiotics.

3. ____ Condoms can reduce the chances of being infected or transmitting some sexually transmitted infections.

4. ____ Gonorrhea can cause sterility.

5. ____ Symptoms of chlamydia include yellow or white discharge from the penis or vagina and a burning sensation during urination.

6. ____ Syphilis is caused by bacteria.

7. ____ Most women infected with gonorrhea show many early symptoms.

8. ____ Benign prostatic hypertrophy is a fairly common disorder that occurs in both women and men as they age.

9. ____ Sexually transmitted infections can be transmitted through contact of the mouth with the genitals of an infected person.

10. ____ Genital HPV infection can be cured with a strong antibiotic.

8. Describe common diseases and disorders of the immune and lymphatic systems

True or False

1. ____ Human immunodeficiency virus (HIV) and acquired immune deficiency syndrome (AIDS) are the same illness.

2. ____ HIV can only be transmitted through sexual contact.

3. ____ The first stage of HIV infection involves symptoms similar to flu.

4. ____ There is no known cure for AIDS.

5. ____ AIDS dementia complex occurs in the early stages of AIDS.

Multiple Choice

6. Care for a person who has HIV or AIDS should focus on
   (A) Helping to find a cure for HIV
   (B) Preventing visits from friends and family so as not to infect them
   (C) Providing relief of symptoms and preventing infection
   (D) Letting the person know that his life choices caused this disease

7. If a resident with AIDS has a poor appetite, the nursing assistant (NA) should
   (A) Give the resident an over-the-counter appetite stimulant
   (B) Serve familiar and favorite foods
   (C) Let the resident know that if he does not eat, he might die
   (D) Discuss this with the resident's friends and family and see what they recommend doing

8. Residents who have AIDS and have infections of the mouth and esophagus may need to eat food that is
   (A) Spicy
   (B) Low in acid
   (C) Dry
   (D) Very hot

9. A resident with AIDS who has nausea and vomiting should
   (A) Eat mostly dairy products
   (B) Eat high-fat foods
   (C) Drink liquids and eat salty foods
   (D) Reduce liquid intake

10. Fluids are important for residents who have diarrhea because
    (A) Diarrhea rapidly depletes the body of fluids
    (B) Diarrhea can be prevented by drinking a lot of fluids
    (C) Diarrhea is an infection that can be flushed out by fluids
    (D) Diarrhea can make a resident's throat dry

11. The following is helpful in dealing with neuropathy (numbness, tingling, and pain in the feet):
(A) Wrapping feet in elastic bandages
(B) Wearing narrow, closed shoes
(C) Using a bed cradle
(D) Tucking in sheets tightly

12. Legal rights regarding HIV or AIDS include
(A) A person with HIV can be fired if the employer did not know that information before the person was hired.
(B) An employer can share an employee's HIV test results with the employee's family members.
(C) A nursing assistant can share a resident's diagnosis of AIDS with anyone the resident may come into contact with.
(D) HIV test results are confidential and cannot be shared with anyone.

Short Answer
Mark an X beside the American Cancer Society's warning signs of cancer.

13. _____ Change in bowel or bladder function

14. _____ Difficulty breathing

15. _____ Dizziness

16. _____ Thickening or lump in breast

17. _____ Memory loss

18. _____ Change in appearance of wart or mole

19. _____ Joint aches

20. _____ Nagging cough

21. _____ Indigestion or difficulty swallowing

22. _____ Nausea

23. _____ Sweet, fruity breath odor

24. _____ Sore that does not heal

25. _____ Unusual bleeding or discharge

26. _____ Headache

Multiple Choice

27. The key treatment for malignant tumors of the skin, breast, bladder, colon, rectum, stomach, and muscle is
(A) Surgery
(B) Homeopathic pills
(C) Radiation
(D) Herbal remedies

28. Nausea, vomiting, diarrhea, hair loss, and decreased resistance to infection are all side effects of which treatment?
(A) Surgery
(B) Chemotherapy
(C) Cold applications
(D) Herbal remedies

29. This treatment method uses medications intravenously to destroy cancer cells and limit the rate of cell growth:
(A) Surgery
(B) Chemotherapy
(C) Radiation
(D) Herbal remedies

30. This treatment method involves removing as much of the tumor as possible to prevent cancer from spreading:
(A) Surgery
(B) Chemotherapy
(C) Radiation
(D) Herbal remedies

31. This treatment method kills normal and abnormal cells in a limited area, sometimes causing skin to become sore, irritated, or burned:
(A) Surgery
(B) Chemotherapy
(C) Radiation
(D) Herbal remedies

32. To help promote proper nutrition for a resident with cancer, the nursing assistant should do the following:
(A) Use metal utensils when serving meals
(B) Serve favorite foods that are high in nutrition
(C) Restrict nutritional supplements
(D) Serve foods with little nutritional content

33. If a resident is experiencing pain, the nursing assistant should
    (A) Assist with comfort measures
    (B) Let the resident know there is little that the NA can do
    (C) Prescribe pain medication
    (D) Give the resident a shot of pain medication

34. Which of the following would be the best response by the NA if a resident with cancer expresses fear and concern about her condition?
    (A) "I know exactly what you're going through because my mother had the same condition."
    (B) "I've read about a new medication that helps cancer like yours."
    (C) "You'll be feeling better in no time."
    (D) "I understand you're scared. Do you feel like talking?"

9. Identify community resources for residents who are ill

Short Answer

1. List three types of organizations that provide services and support for people who are ill and their families.

   _____

   _____

   _____

   _____

   _____

   _____

Name: _____

19

Confusion, Dementia, and Alzheimer's Disease

1. Describe normal changes of aging in the brain

Multiple Choice

1. The loss of ability to think logically and clearly is called
   (A) Cognitive impairment
   (B) Cerebrovascular obstruction
   (C) Cardiovascular loss
   (D) Developmental disability

2. Cognitive impairment affects
   (A) Respiratory rate
   (B) Motor skills
   (C) Concentration and memory
   (D) Diet and exercise

3. Nursing assistants can help elderly residents with memory loss by
   (A) Doing as much as possible for them
   (B) Encouraging them to make lists of things to remember
   (C) Reminding them every time they forget something
   (D) Telling them to think as hard as they can

2. Discuss confusion and delirium

Short Answer

1. What are ten actions that a nursing assistant can take when helping care for a resident who is confused?

_____

_____

_____

_____

_____

_____

_____

_____

_____

_____

_____

_____

_____

_____

_____

_____

2. Name four possible causes of delirium.

_____

_____

_____

_____

3. Describe dementia and define related terms

True or False

1. _____ Dementia is the loss of mental abilities such as thinking, remembering, reasoning, and communicating.

2. _____ Dementia is something that happens as every person gets older.

3. _____ An irreversible disease can usually be cured with medication and/or surgery.

4. _____ Degenerative diseases get continually worse, causing a greater loss of health and abilities.

Name: _____

5. _____ Parkinson's disease may cause dementia.

4. Describe Alzheimer's disease and identify its stages

True or False

1. _____ Alzheimer's disease is the most common cause of dementia in the elderly.

2. _____ Men are more likely to have Alzheimer's disease than women.

3. _____ Alzheimer's disease is a normal part of aging, and everyone will develop it at some point in their lives.

4. _____ Alzheimer's disease causes tangled nerve fibers and protein deposits to form in the brain, eventually causing dementia.

5. _____ There is no cure for Alzheimer's disease.

6. _____ There is one simple exam that is performed to diagnose Alzheimer's disease.

7. _____ Symptoms of Alzheimer's disease typically appear suddenly.

8. _____ Each person with Alzheimer's disease will show different signs at different times.

9. _____ Skills that a person has learned recently are usually kept longer after the onset of Alzheimer's disease.

10. _____ Eventually most Alzheimer's disease victims will be dependent on others for care.

11. _____ Generally speaking, middle-stage Alzheimer's disease lasts the longest out of the three stages.

12. _____ Once a resident is in late-stage Alzheimer's disease, the nursing assistant should no longer encourage independence.

5. Identify personal attitudes helpful in caring for residents with Alzheimer's disease

Scenarios
Read each scenario below. State which of the personal attitudes from the learning objective would be helpful in each situation and explain why.

1. An NA has been working all day and is very tired. He has a headache and has not had time to eat a decent meal. He does not know how he will summon the energy to come back to work tomorrow and take care of Mrs. Jones, a resident with Alzheimer's disease whose behavior has been very challenging lately.

_____

_____

_____

_____

_____

_____

_____

_____

2. Ms. Yancy has Alzheimer's disease. She is still in the very early stages of the disease, but she gets very depressed when she thinks about what will happen to her later. She has not opened up to her NA about things that she likes to do or talk about, and the NA would like her to be more comfortable with her. She notices that when Ms. Yancy's daughter visits, she always brightens up a bit.

_____

_____

_____

_____

_____

_____

3. A resident becomes very depressed one morning while his NA is helping him shave. He tells the NA she is lucky that she does not need someone to help her do everyday tasks. He says that he hopes she appreciates her good health.

_____

_____

_____

_____

_____

_____

4. A resident tells an NA that she hates having to see him every morning. She says that she does not know how anyone was foolish enough to hire him and that she will be complaining to the nurse about him every day until he is fired.

_____

_____

_____

_____

_____

_____

5. On Monday afternoon, Mr. Kotter was lively and friendly. He said that he was looking forward to a Tuesday afternoon card game that he was going to have with his two best friends. On Tuesday when an NA stops by his room to get him ready to go to the card game, he says he hates cards and he does not like any of the people who are playing. He would prefer to go for a walk by himself.

_____

_____

_____

_____

_____

_____

6. List strategies for better communication with residents with Alzheimer's disease

Scenarios
Read each scenario below and state an appropriate response.

1. Mrs. Hays, a resident with Alzheimer's disease, has awakened from her nap and does not recognize her room or anyone around her.

_____

_____

_____

_____

_____

2. Blake, an NA, has been trying to give Mr. Collins, a resident with Alzheimer's disease, a bath. Mr. Collins has become agitated and is asking Blake, "Who are you?" over and over again, although Blake has already identified himself twice.

_____

_____

_____

_____

_____

3. Mrs. Hays has been telling Blake a story about her niece. She is showing him a necklace that her niece had given her as a gift. She is having trouble remembering the word necklace and is getting upset.

_____

_____

_____

_____

_____

_____

4. Blake is helping Mr. Collins get ready to go to dinner. Blake asks him to put his shoes on, but Mr. Collins does not understand what Blake wants him to do.

_____

_____

_____

_____

_____

_____

Multiple Choice

5. When communicating with a resident with Alzheimer's disease, the NA should
   (A) Quietly approach the resident from behind
   (B) Stand as close as possible to the resident
   (C) Communicate in a loud, busy place to help cheer up the resident
   (D) Speak slowly, using a lower tone of voice than normal

6. If a resident is frightened or anxious, which of the following should the NA do?
   (A) Check her body language so she does not appear tense or hurried
   (B) Turn up the television or radio to try to distract the resident
   (C) Use complex, longer sentences to calm the resident
   (D) Give multiple instructions at one time so that the resident has time to understand them

7. If a resident perseverates, this means he is
   (A) Repeating words, phrases, questions, or actions
   (B) Suggesting words that sound correct
   (C) Hallucinating or having delusions
   (D) Gesturing instead of speaking

8. If a resident does not remember how to perform basic tasks, the NA should
   (A) Do everything for him
   (B) Encourage the resident to do what he can
   (C) Skip explaining each activity
   (D) Say "don't" as often as the NA feels is necessary

9. If a resident repeatedly asks if he can go home, the NA should
   (A) Let the resident know he can never go home due to having Alzheimer's disease
   (B) Ask the resident to talk about what his home was like
   (C) Nicely ask the resident to stop asking that question
   (D) Tell the resident that he can go home when his condition improves

7. Explain general principles that will help assist residents with personal care

Fill in the Blank
Fill in the blanks below for guidelines that nursing assistants should follow when assisting residents with Alzheimer's disease.

1. Develop a _____ and stick to it.

2. Being _____ is important for residents who are confused and easily upset.

3. Promote _____. This will help residents _____ with a difficult disease like Alzheimer's disease.

4. Take care of yourself, both

_____ and physically.

8. List and describe interventions for problems with common activities of daily living (ADLs)

Short Answer
For each of the following statements, write good idea *if the statement is a good idea for residents with Alzheimer's disease or* bad idea *if the statement is a bad idea.*

1. Use nonslip mats, tub seats, and handholds to ensure safety during bathing.

   _____

2. Always bathe the resident at the same time every day, even if she is agitated.

   _____

3. Break tasks down into simple steps, explaining one step at a time.

   _____

4. Do not attempt to groom the resident; he most likely does not care about his appearance anyway.

   _____

5. Choose clothes that are simple to put on.

   _____

6. If the resident is incontinent, do not give him fluids because it makes the problem worse.

   _____

7. Mark the bathroom with a sign or picture as a reminder of when to use it and where it is.

   _____

8. Check the skin regularly for signs of irritation.

   _____

9. Follow Standard Precautions when caring for the resident.

   _____

10. Do not encourage exercise, as this will make the resident more agitated.

    _____

11. Serve finger foods if the resident tends to wander during meals.

    _____

12. Schedule meals at the same time every day.

    _____

13. Serve new kinds of foods as often as possible to stimulate the resident.

    _____

14. Put only one kind of food on the plate at a time.

    _____

15. Use plain white dishes for serving food.

    _____

16. Do not encourage independence, as this can lead to aggressive behavior.

    _____

17. Protect privacy by keeping the resident covered, even if he is unaware of what is happening.

    _____

18. Reward positive behavior with smiles and warm touches.

    _____

9. List and describe interventions for common difficult behaviors related to Alzheimer's disease

Scenarios
For each description below, identify the behavior that the resident with Alzheimer's disease is exhibiting and describe one way of dealing with it.

1. Mrs. Donne gets upset at about 9:00 p.m. every night. She repeatedly asks for snacks or drinks and refuses to go to bed.

   _____

   _____

   _____

   _____

   _____

Name: _____

2. Mr. Noble is playing chess with a friend and becomes angry when he loses the game. He shoves his friend, and when the nursing assistant approaches them, he tells her he is going to hit her.

_____

_____

_____

_____

_____

3. Mrs. Martin gets very upset every time she sees the president on television. She yells at the screen and tells everyone what a poor state our country is in.

_____

_____

_____

_____

_____

_____

4. Ms. Desmond used to enjoy talking to people and reading, but lately she does not seem to enjoy anything. She sleeps most of the day and never talks to anyone unless she is asked to.

_____

_____

_____

_____

_____

_____

5. Whenever Mr. Henderson does not like what is being served for dinner, he bangs on the table with his fists and shouts about how

much he hates his food. When people try to get him to stop, he only seems to grow louder.

_____

_____

_____

_____

_____

_____

6. Ms. Storey is walking around the facility asking everyone she meets what time it is. Even though she has been told several times, she still seems unsatisfied and keeps asking the question.

_____

_____

_____

_____

_____

_____

7. About an hour before dinner every night, Ms. Lordes starts walking up and down the hall as quickly as she can. She does not speak to or acknowledge anyone else while she is doing this.

_____

_____

_____

_____

_____

_____

8. Whenever a female resident comes into the television room, Mr. Radcliffe tells her that he loves her and starts removing his clothes. If she stays in the room long enough, he will ask her to take off her clothes, too.

_____

_____

_____

_____

_____

9. Mrs. Leone loves the color red. She has a lot of red clothing that she enjoys wearing. Whenever she sees a piece of red clothing, even in another resident's room, she picks it up and takes it back to her room.

_____

_____

_____

_____

_____

_____

10. Mr. Montoya tells his nursing assistant that his wife has just called him on the phone. She is coming to pick him up, and they are going to dinner at the place they went on their first date. The NA knows that his wife has been dead for several years, and their favorite restaurant has long since closed down.

_____

_____

_____

_____

_____

_____

_____

10. Describe creative therapies for residents with Alzheimer's disease

Scenarios

For each situation described below, identify the therapy that the nursing assistant is using.

1. Ms. Lee misses her husband, who has been dead for ten years, very much. Lisa, an NA who works with her, always asks about her life with her husband and what it was like. Ms. Lee seems to enjoy telling Lisa stories about what they did when they were young and how happy she was when they were together.

_____

_____

2. Mr. Elking tells Lisa that he has a date with Nora, the pretty girl who lives across the street. He is going to take her dancing and out to a movie. Lisa knows that Nora lived in his neighborhood when he was a teenager and he has not seen her for years. She also knows that Mr. Elking rarely gets out of bed. Instead of correcting him, Lisa asks him what kind of movie they are going to see and what he thinks he should wear.

_____

_____

3. Mr. Tennant sometimes gets depressed, especially in the evenings. Lisa knows that he loves classical music, so she starts playing it for him in the evenings a little before he usually starts feeling sad. He sorts through albums and places them in stacks.

_____

_____

11. Discuss how Alzheimer's disease may affect the family

Short Answer

1. Why might it be difficult for families of people who have AD?

_____

_____

_____

_____

_____

_____

2. What two major resources affect the ability of a resident's family to cope with AD?

_____

_____

_____

_____

_____

12. Identify community resources available to people with Alzheimer's disease and their families

Short Answer

1. List four resources available to people with Alzheimer's disease and their families.

_____

_____

_____

_____

_____

_____

20

Mental Health and Mental Illness

1. Identify seven characteristics of mental health

Short Answer

1. Define mental health.

    _____

    _____

    _____

    _____

    _____

2. List seven characteristics of a person who is mentally healthy.

    _____

    _____

    _____

    _____

    _____

    _____

    _____

    _____

    _____

    _____

2. Identify four causes of mental illness

True or False

1. _____   Signs and symptoms of mental illness include confusion, disorientation, agitation, and anxiety.

2. _____   A situation response may be triggered by severe changes in the environment.

3. _____   A person who is mentally healthy cannot experience a situation response.

4. _____   Mental illness can be caused by substance abuse or a chemical imbalance.

5. _____   The building blocks of mental health are self-respect and self-worth.

6. _____   Traumatic experiences early in life do not cause mental illness.

7. _____   Mental illness cannot be inherited.

8. _____   Extreme stress may result in mental illness.

9. _____   Mental illness is a disorder.

3. Distinguish between fact and fallacy concerning mental illness

True or False

1. _____   A fallacy is a false belief.

2. _____   People who have a mental illness have the power to control their illness if they really want to.

3. _____   People who have a mental illness usually do not want to get well.

4. _____   Mental illness is a disorder just like any physical illness.

5. _____   People who are mentally ill often cannot control their emotions or responses.

6. _____   An intellectual disability is a type of mental illness.

4. Explain the connection between mental and physical wellness

Short Answer

1. Briefly describe why mental health is important to physical health.

_____

_____

_____

_____

_____

_____

_____

_____

_____

_____

_____

5. List guidelines for communicating with residents who are mentally ill

Short Answer

1. When communicating with a resident who has a mental illness, why is it important for the nursing assistant to treat each resident as an individual and to tailor the NA's style of communication to the situation?

_____

_____

_____

_____

_____

_____

2. When communicating with a resident who has a mental illness, why is it important for the nursing assistant not to talk to him as if he were a child?

_____

_____

_____

_____

6. Identify and define common defense mechanisms

Short Answer
Read each description below and identify the defense mechanism that is being used.

1. When Aaron's mother yells at him for breaking a vase in the living room, he goes into his room and yells at his stuffed bear.

_____

_____

_____

2. When Gia was 10, she was very badly injured in a car accident. She was in the hospital for almost three months, but now she tries not to think about that time.

_____

_____

_____

3. When Mark accuses his little sister Sarah of having a crush on the boy who sits next to her in class, she blushes and cries, "I do not!"

_____

_____

_____

4. When Esther was 42, her husband died of lung cancer. After his death, she got out the quilt she used to sleep with as a child and curled up in bed with it for days.

_____

_____

5. Wayne is fixing a leaky sink in the bathroom. When his wife teases him about taking a long time to fix it, he replies, "It's not my fault. I can't concentrate on anything with you bothering me all the time."

_____
_____
_____
_____

6. Martin's girlfriend promised to go out with him on Thursday night, but she forgot and made plans with her sister instead. Martin is annoyed, but does not say anything to her. When he goes out with his friends that night, he tells them that she is mad at him.

_____
_____
_____
_____

7. Describe anxiety, depression, and schizophrenia

Multiple Choice

1. Uneasiness, worry, or fear, often about a situation or condition, is called
    (A) Anxiety
    (B) Withdrawal
    (C) Fatigue
    (D) Apathy

2. An intense, irrational fear of an object, place, or situation is called a
    (A) Depressive episode
    (B) Delusion
    (C) Phobia
    (D) Hallucination

3. Which type of mental illness is most commonly associated with suicide in older adults?
    (A) Anxiety
    (B) Apathy
    (C) Irritability
    (D) Depression

4. Which of the following means a lack of interest in activities?
    (A) Guilt
    (B) Depression
    (C) Apathy
    (D) Delusion

5. A persistent false belief, such as a person believing that someone else is controlling his thoughts, is a
    (A) Defense mechanism
    (B) Delusion
    (C) Phobia
    (D) Hallucination

8. Explain how mental illness is treated

True or False

1. _____ Mental illness cannot be treated.

2. _____ Medication and psychotherapy are commonly used to treat mental illness.

3. _____ Nursing assistants are responsible for giving residents their medication for depression.

4. _____ Cognitive behavioral therapy is often used to treat anxiety.

9. Explain the nursing assistant's role in caring for residents who are mentally ill

Short Answer

1. List three special responsibilities that nursing assistants have when caring for residents who have a mental illness.

_____
_____
_____
_____
_____
_____
_____

2. List three responsibilities that home health aides may have when working with clients who have a mental illness.

_____

_____

_____

_____

_____

_____

_____

10. Identify important observations that should be made and reported

True or False

1. _____ It is important for the nursing assistant to report to the nurse if a resident stops taking his medication.

2. _____ As long as a resident is joking when talking about suicide, the nursing assistant does not need to report it.

11. List the signs of substance abuse

Multiple Choice

1. Circle any of the following substances that can be abused:
   (A) Alcohol
   (B) Cigarettes
   (C) Decongestants
   (D) Diet aids
   (E) Illegal drugs
   (F) Glue
   (G) Paint
   (H) Prescription medicine

2. A resident has been acting a little strangely lately. She gets upset very easily, and her eyes are always red. She does not eat much, and sometimes her nursing assistant can smell alcohol on her breath, even in the morning. What would be the best response by the NA?
   (A) Confront the resident about what the NA has noticed
   (B) Call Alcoholics Anonymous to get advice on how to handle the situation
   (C) Document the NA's observations and report them to the nurse
   (D) Search the resident's dresser and side table for alcohol and throw away any alcohol found

21

Rehabilitation and Restorative Care

1. Discuss rehabilitation and restorative care

Multiple Choice

1. What is the goal of rehabilitation?
   (A) To diagnose a disease
   (B) To restore the person to the highest possible level of functioning
   (C) To reach the level of functionality of a normal person
   (D) To cure a disease

2. Which care team member establishes the goals of care for rehabilitation?
   (A) Doctor
   (B) Social worker
   (C) Nursing assistant
   (D) Counselor

3. What is the goal of restorative care?
   (A) To diagnose new diseases
   (B) To create new infection prevention policies
   (C) To keep the resident at the level achieved by rehabilitation
   (D) To get the family to visit more often

Short Answer

4. Rehabilitation will be used for many residents, but particularly for those who have suffered what incidents?

   _____

   _____

   _____

   _____

   _____

5. Why are nursing assistants a very important part of the restorative care team?

   _____

   _____

   _____

   _____

   _____

   _____

   _____

   _____

True or False

6. _____ The nursing assistant should ignore any setbacks a resident experiences so she does not become discouraged.

7. _____ All residents will enjoy being encouraged in an obvious way.

8. _____ The nursing assistant should do everything for the resident, rather than having him try to do it himself. Doing this will help speed recovery.

9. _____ The NA should not report any decline in a resident's ability because all residents in restorative care will have a decline in ability.

10. _____ Family members and residents will take cues from the nursing assistant on how to behave.

11. _____ Tasks should be broken down into small steps.

12. _____ It is important for the NA to report any signs of depression or mood changes in a resident.

13. _____ When a resident is demanding or irritating, the NA can unplug his call light until his attitude improves.

2. Describe the importance of promoting independence and list ways that exercise improves health

Short Answer

1. List nine problems that can result from inactivity and immobility.

    _____

    _____

    _____

    _____

    _____

    _____

    _____

    _____

    _____

2. What do regular ambulation and exercise help improve?

    _____

    _____

    _____

    _____

    _____

3. Describe assistive devices and equipment

Multiple Choice

1. Assistive devices help residents
    (A) Fight infection
    (B) Make decisions about care
    (C) Perform their activities of daily living
    (D) Communicate

2. Supportive devices are used to assist residents with
    (A) Personal care
    (B) Ambulation
    (C) Burns
    (D) Vital signs

3. Safety devices are used for
    (A) Preventing accidents
    (B) Sleeping
    (C) Ambulation
    (D) Incontinence

Short Answer

4. Choose an adaptive device from Figure 21-4 in the textbook that you did not choose for the Chapter Review. Describe how it might help a resident who is recovering from or adapting to a physical condition.

    _____

    _____

    _____

    _____

    _____

4. Explain guidelines for maintaining proper body alignment

Fill in the Blank

1. Observe principles of

    _____. Remember that proper alignment is based on a straight

    _____.

    _____ or rolled or folded _____ may be needed to support the small of the back and raise the knees or head in the supine position.

2. Keep body parts in natural

    _____.

    In a natural hand position, the fingers are slightly _____.
    Use _____ to keep covers from resting on feet in the supine position.

3. Prevent external rotation of

    _____. Change _____ frequently to prevent muscle stiffness and pressure injuries. This should be done at least every _____ hours.

5. Explain care guidelines for prosthetic devices

True or False

1. ____ When cleaning the eye after an artificial eye is removed, the nursing assistant should wipe gently from the outer area toward the inner area.

2. ____ Prostheses are relatively inexpensive and are easy to replace.

3. ____ Artificial eyes are held in place by a special type of glue.

4. ____ A prosthesis is a device that replaces a body part that is missing or deformed because of an accident, injury, illness, or birth defect.

5. ____ Artificial eyes should be rinsed in rubbing alcohol to prevent infection.

6. ____ If a prosthesis is broken, it is best for the NA to try to repair it before bothering the nurse about it.

7. ____ When observing the skin on the stump, it is important that the NA check for signs of skin breakdown caused by pressure and abrasion.

6. Describe how to assist with range of motion exercises

Matching
Use each letter only once.

1. ____ Active assisted range of motion (AAROM)

2. ____ Active range of motion (AROM)

3. ____ Passive range of motion (PROM)

4. ____ Range of motion (ROM)

(A) Exercises performed by the resident with some assistance and support

(B) Exercises used by residents who are not able to move on their own

(C) Exercises that put a particular joint through its full arc of motion

(D) Exercises performed by the resident himself, without help

Labeling
For each of the following illustrations, write the correct term for each body movement.

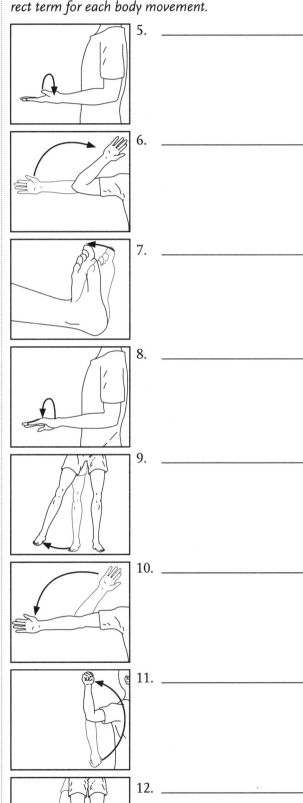

5. _____

6. _____

7. _____

8. _____

9. _____

10. _____

11. _____

12. _____

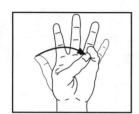 13. _____

Multiple Choice

14. In what order should the NA perform range of motion exercises?
    (A) He should start from the feet and work upward.
    (B) He should start from the shoulders and work downward.
    (C) He should start at the hands and work inward.
    (D) He should exercise the arms last.

15. If a resident reports pain during range of motion exercises, the NA should
    (A) Continue with the exercises as planned
    (B) Continue, but perform the motion that caused pain more gently
    (C) Stop the exercises and report the pain to the nurse
    (D) Stop the motion for one minute before starting again

16. How many times should each range of motion exercise be repeated?
    (A) At least 6 times
    (B) At least 10 times
    (C) At least 12 times
    (D) At least 3 times

7. Describe the benefits of deep breathing exercises

Short Answer

1. What can deep breathing exercises help?

    _____

    _____

    _____

    _____

    _____

    _____

22

Special Care Skills

1. Understand the types of residents who are in a subacute setting

True or False

1. _____ A subacute setting is a special unit for those who need more care than most long-term facilities can give.

2. _____ Hospitals can provide subacute care, but skilled nursing facilities cannot.

3. _____ People who have had surgery, have chronic illnesses, or require dialysis or complex wound care may need subacute care.

4. _____ A mechanical ventilator is a machine that assists with or replaces breathing when a person cannot breathe on his own.

2. Discuss reasons for and types of surgery

Multiple Choice

1. Which type of surgery must be performed for health reasons, but is not an emergency?
   (A) Elective
   (B) Urgent
   (C) Emergency
   (D) Plastic

2. _____ surgery is unexpected and unscheduled and must be performed immediately to save a life or limb.
   (A) Elective
   (B) Urgent
   (C) Emergency
   (D) Plastic

3. Which type of surgery is chosen by the patient and is planned in advance?
   (A) Elective
   (B) Urgent
   (C) Emergency
   (D) Non-elective

4. Which type of anesthesia is injected directly into the surgical site or area and is used for minor surgical procedures?
   (A) Local anesthesia
   (B) General anesthesia
   (C) Full body anesthesia
   (D) Intravenous anesthesia

5. An epidural is an example of this type of anesthesia:
   (A) Regional anesthesia
   (B) General anesthesia
   (C) Local anesthesia
   (D) Intravenous anesthesia

3. Discuss preoperative care

True or False

1. _____ Before a person has surgery, the doctor will most likely not tell him what to expect because it may frighten the person too much.

2. _____ People who are going to have surgery often experience anxiety, fear, worry, and sadness.

3. _____ A nursing assistant can help a person who is worried about surgery by avoiding the person until the surgery is over.

4. _____ If a person has an *NPO* medical order before surgery, this means that she cannot have food or anything to drink except for water.

5. ____ A nursing assistant's duties may include making sure that the person's identification bracelet is accurate and on the wrist or ankle prior to transport.

4. Describe postoperative care

Short Answer

1. What are three goals of postoperative care?

    _____

    _____

    _____

    _____

2. What are the concerns and possible complications to watch for after a person has surgery?

    _____

    _____

    _____

    _____

3. What type of equipment might a nursing assistant be asked to gather while a resident is in recovery after surgery?

    _____

    _____

    _____

    _____

4. List ten postoperative care tasks that nursing assistants may be required to do.

    _____

    _____

    _____

    _____

    _____

    _____

    _____

    _____

    _____

_____

_____

_____

_____

_____

5. List care guidelines for pulse oximetry

Multiple Choice

1. Pulse oximetry is commonly used for people who are
    (A) Diabetic
    (B) Incontinent
    (C) Returning from surgery
    (D) Demented

2. A pulse oximeter measures
    (A) Blood oxygen level
    (B) Swelling of the extremities
    (C) Weight
    (D) Medication levels

3. The pulse oximeter's sensor is usually clipped on a person's
    (A) Knee
    (B) Elbow
    (C) Chin
    (D) Finger

4. The sensor uses _____ to measure blood oxygen level.
    (A) Light
    (B) Sound
    (C) Chemicals
    (D) Vibrations

5. A normal blood oxygen level is usually between
    (A) 25% - 40%
    (B) 40% - 60%
    (C) 60% - 70%
    (D) 95% - 100%

6. Which of the following should be reported to the nurse regarding pulse oximetry?
    (A) The oximeter displays the blood oxygen level.
    (B) The oximeter displays the person's pulse rate.
    (C) The alarm sounds.
    (D) The resident requests extra pillows.

6. Describe telemetry and list care guidelines

Fill in the Blank

1. Telemetry is used to measure the heart _____ and _____ on a continuous basis.

2. Wires are attached to the _____ with sticky pads or patches.

3. The nursing assistant should report to the nurse if the pads become _____ or soiled.

4. If the _____ sounds, the NA should notify the nurse.

5. The NA should check _____ signs as ordered.

6. The skin around the pads should be checked for sores, redness, or _____.

7. Explain artificial airways and list care guidelines

Short Answer

1. List three situations in which an artificial airway might be necessary.

_____

_____

_____

_____

2. What is a tracheostomy?

_____

_____

_____

_____

3. List four guidelines for nursing assistants working with residents who have artificial airways.

_____

_____

_____

_____

_____

8. Discuss care for a resident with a tracheostomy

True or False

1. _____ A tracheostomy is always permanent.

2. _____ It may be difficult for the resident to talk after first having a tracheostomy placed.

3. _____ Cancer, infection, and severe neck or mouth injuries are some reasons why a tracheostomy may be necessary.

4. _____ Gurgling sounds are normal due to the placement in the neck and do not need to be reported to the nurse.

5. _____ Nursing assistants do not perform tracheostomy care or suctioning.

6. _____ Shortness of breath or trouble breathing should be reported right away.

7. _____ Residents with tracheostomies are prone to respiratory infections.

8. _____ To help prevent infection when working with residents with tracheostomies, the nursing assistant should wash his hands often.

9. List care guidelines for residents requiring mechanical ventilation

Crossword

Across

3. Being on a ventilator has been compared to breathing through this

4. Nursing assistants should answer these promptly

6. An agent or drug that helps calm and soothe a person

Down

1. Regular, careful skin care can prevent these types of wounds

2. Something that a person will no longer be able to do while on the mechanical ventilator because air will no longer reach the larynx

5. Mechanical ventilation inflates and deflates these

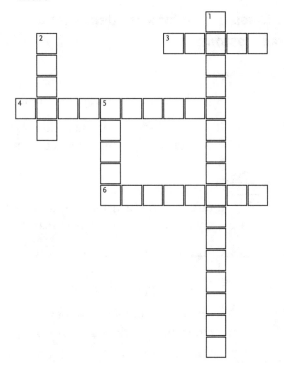

10. Describe suctioning and list signs of respiratory distress

True or False

1. ____ Suctioning is needed when a person cannot remove mucus and secretions from the lungs on his own.

2. ____ Suctioning is usually a non-sterile procedure.

3. ____ The nursing assistant is normally responsible for suctioning.

4. ____ A portable pump may be used to suction the resident.

5. ____ One sign of respiratory distress is a gurgling sound of secretions.

6. ____ If a person is flaring his nostrils, he may be in respiratory distress.

7. ____ Vital signs, especially respiratory rate, should be monitored closely.

11. Describe chest tubes and explain related care

Multiple Choice

1. Chest tubes are inserted during a _____ procedure.
   (A) Sterile
   (B) Non-sterile
   (C) Personal care
   (D) Catheterized

2. Chest tubes drain air, blood, or fluid from
   (A) The heart
   (B) The brain
   (C) The pleural cavity
   (D) The esophagus

3. Chest tubes may be required for
   (A) Vaginitis
   (B) Eczema
   (C) Nutritional deficiencies
   (D) Trauma

4. The drainage system must be
   (A) Recycled
   (B) Permanent
   (C) Airtight
   (D) Frozen

5. The drainage system must be kept _____ the level of the resident's chest.
   (A) Above
   (B) Below
   (C) Beside
   (D) Equal distance to

23

Dying, Death, and Hospice

1. Discuss the stages of grief

True or False

1. _____ A terminal illness will eventually cause death.

2. _____ Older people or those with terminal illnesses rarely have time to prepare for death.

3. _____ Preparing for death is a process that affects the dying person's emotions and behavior.

4. _____ All people with terminal illnesses will pass through each stage described by Dr. Kübler-Ross.

5. _____ Residents may move back and forth between the stages of the grief process.

Multiple Choice

Read each scenario below and choose which stage of grief the person described is experiencing.

6. Mr. Cane was told two years ago that a tumor in his brain was inoperable and would eventually be fatal. Since that time, he has visited many specialists. Despite receiving the same diagnosis from every doctor, he continues to seek further opinions, insisting that each doctor try to remove the tumor. Which stage of grief is Mr. Cane in?
   (A) Denial
   (B) Anger
   (C) Bargaining
   (D) Depression
   (E) Acceptance

7. Mrs. Tyler is dying of heart disease. One day as her nursing assistant, Annie, is assisting her with personal care, Mrs. Tyler lashes out at her. She tells Annie that she is a dumb girl who is wasting her life and does not deserve the many years she has left to live. Which stage of grief is Mrs. Tyler in?
   (A) Denial
   (B) Anger
   (C) Bargaining
   (D) Depression
   (E) Acceptance

8. Mr. Lopez is dying of AIDS. He has called all of his friends to say goodbye and has discussed at length with his family the kind of memorial service he would like them to arrange. What stage of grief is Mr. Lopez in?
   (A) Denial
   (B) Anger
   (C) Bargaining
   (D) Depression
   (E) Acceptance

9. Ms. Corke has always been lively and happy. Since she learned that she has Lou Gehrig's disease, however, her mood has changed drastically. Although she is still healthy enough to do activities, she rarely leaves her room or even changes out of her nightclothes. Which stage of grief is Ms. Corke in?
   (A) Denial
   (B) Anger
   (C) Bargaining
   (D) Depression
   (E) Acceptance

10. Mrs. Palmer has terminal cancer. When her children try to talk to her about what kind of arrangements she wants to make for finances and her funeral, she seems not to know what they are talking about. She talks about making plans to take her granddaughter on a trip to Europe after her graduation. Which stage of grief is Mrs. Palmer in?
    (A) Denial
    (B) Anger
    (C) Bargaining
    (D) Depression
    (E) Acceptance

11. Mr. Celasco has had lung cancer for several years. During that time, he has tried to quit smoking but has been unsuccessful. When he finds out that there are no further treatments for him to try, he pledges that he will give up smoking in exchange for a few more years of life. What stage of grief is Mr. Celasco in?
    (A) Denial
    (B) Anger
    (C) Bargaining
    (D) Depression
    (E) Acceptance

12. Mr. Jansen suffers from Alzheimer's disease. He knows that eventually he will die from the disease and that, before then, he will become incapable of making decisions regarding his estate. He contacts his lawyer to arrange things while he still has time to make competent decisions himself. Which stage of grief is Mr. Jansen in?
    (A) Denial
    (B) Anger
    (C) Bargaining
    (D) Depression
    (E) Acceptance

2. Describe the grief process

Multiple Choice
Read each scenario below and choose the reaction to a loved one's death that each person is experiencing.

1. Malcolm's wife died during the birth of their second daughter. Malcolm is so upset with her for abandoning him and the children that he cannot even stand to hear her name spoken. What reaction is Malcolm experiencing?
    (A) Loneliness
    (B) Denial
    (C) Anger
    (D) Guilt
    (E) Sadness

2. Becky's mother had been ill for many years before she died when Becky was 15 years old. After her death, Becky remembers how she used to resent helping her mother around the house so much and wishes that she had been kinder and more cheerful. Which reaction is she having?
    (A) Anger
    (B) Sadness
    (C) Guilt
    (D) Denial
    (E) Relief

3. Melinda's grandmother, to whom she was very close, died of a long illness on Sunday afternoon. On Monday morning, Melinda's mother is astonished to find Melinda getting ready for school as she does every Monday morning. Which reaction is Melinda having?
    (A) Loneliness
    (B) Denial
    (C) Relief
    (D) Guilt
    (E) Regret

4. Micah's best friend, Lawrence, died of cancer at the age of 45. Whenever Micah spends time with the friends that they had in common, he is reminded of Lawrence and feels sad. He is not as close to his other friends as he was to Lawrence, and he feels he has no one to confide in with Lawrence gone. Which reaction is he having?
    (A) Shock
    (B) Denial
    (C) Anger
    (D) Loneliness
    (E) Guilt

5. Theresa's 9-year-old son went to a pool party for a friend's birthday and accidentally drowned. Theresa has been unable to forgive herself for letting him go to the party. What reaction is she having?
   (A) Anger
   (B) Loneliness
   (C) Denial
   (D) Guilt
   (E) Shock

6. Casey's brother was killed suddenly in a car accident. He is surprised that he seems to feel very little emotion regarding the death. Which reaction is Casey having?
   (A) Loneliness
   (B) Shock
   (C) Guilt
   (D) Anger
   (E) Regret

7. When Elizabeth's boyfriend was killed by a drunk driver on his way home one night, Elizabeth was inconsolable. She has stopped seeing her friends and stays in her room crying for hours at a time. Which reaction is she having?
   (A) Anger
   (B) Sadness
   (C) Guilt
   (D) Denial
   (E) Regret

8. Marcela's father recently died after battling congestive heart failure for many years. When he got sicker, Marcela had to take a leave of absence from work to help deal with his care, which greatly affected her income and caused her worry. She found herself resenting him at times. After he died, Marcela felt sad, but she also thinks about how she is free to make her own decisions about her life again. Which reaction is she having?
   (A) Anger
   (B) Sadness
   (C) Relief
   (D) Denial
   (E) Regret

3. Discuss how feelings and attitudes about death differ

Short Answer

1. Have you ever experienced the death of a loved one? If so, what are some of the emotions you felt?

_____

_____

_____

_____

_____

_____

_____

_____

_____

_____

2. What, if any, religious or spiritual beliefs do you subscribe to? How do they influence your feelings about death? If you do not have any religious or spiritual beliefs, what are your feelings about death?

_____

_____

_____

_____

_____

_____

_____

_____

_____

_____

3. What cultural background do you have? What cultures are you familiar with? Briefly describe how your culture or other cultures you are familiar with feel about death.

_____

_____

_____

_____

_____

_____

_____

_____

_____

_____

4. Discuss how to care for a resident who is dying

Fill in the Blank

1. _____ perspiring residents often; skin should be clean and dry.

2. Residents may not be able to communicate that they are in

   _____.

   Observe for signs and report them.

3. Changes of position, back massage, skin care, mouth care, and proper body

   _____

   may help relieve pain.

4. _____ may be one of the most important things you can do for a resident who is dying. Pay attention to these conversations.

5. _____ can be very important. Holding your resident's hand can be comforting.

6. Do not

   _____

   the dying person or his family. Do not deny that death is approaching, and do not tell the resident that anyone knows how or when it will happen.

7. _____ is usually the last sense to leave the body.

8. Provide

   _____

   for visits from clergy, family, and friends.

9. Do not discuss your personal

   _____

   or spiritual beliefs with residents or their families or make recommendations.

5. Describe ways to treat dying residents and their families with dignity and how to honor their rights

Short Answer

1. List three legal rights that must be honored when working with residents who are dying.

   _____

   _____

   _____

   _____

   _____

   _____

   _____

   _____

   _____

2. Look at *The Dying Person's Bill of Rights* on page 406 of the textbook. Pick three rights that you feel would be most important to you. Briefly describe why they would be important to you.

   _____

   _____

_____

_____

_____

_____

_____

_____

_____

_____

_____

_____

_____

_____

_____

6. Define the goals of a hospice program

Multiple Choice

1. Hospice care is the term for compassionate care given to
   (A) Residents who have respiratory diseases
   (B) Residents who are dying
   (C) Residents with Parkinson's disease
   (D) Residents with developmental disabilities

2. Hospice care encourages residents to
   (A) Allow hospice care teams to handle all care decisions
   (B) Allow lawyers to make care decisions
   (C) Allow doctors to make care decisions
   (D) Participate in their own care as much as possible

3. Hospice goals focus on
   (A) Recovery of the person
   (B) Comfort and dignity of the person
   (C) Curing disease
   (D) Creating a will and other legal documents for the person

4. Focusing on pain relief, controlling symptoms, and preventing complications is called _____ care.
   (A) Palliative
   (B) Personal
   (C) Professional
   (D) Pediatric

Short Answer

5. List seven guidelines that are helpful for hospice work.

_____

_____

_____

_____

_____

_____

_____

_____

_____

_____

7. Explain common signs of approaching death

Short Answer
Place a check mark (✓) beside the signs of approaching death.

1. _____ High blood pressure

2. _____ Fever

3. _____ Cold, pale skin

4. _____ Disorientation

5. _____ Healthy skin tone

6. _____ Heightened sense of touch

7. _____ Impaired speech

8. _____ Incontinence

9. _____ Perspiration

10. _____ Strong pulse

8. List changes that may occur in the human body after death

True or False

1. ____ When death occurs, the body will not have a heartbeat.

2. ____ The eyelids will automatically close after death.

3. ____ The body may be incontinent of both urine and stool after death.

4. ____ The muscles in the body become loose and relaxed after death.

5. ____ The nurse should be called immediately to confirm death.

9. Describe postmortem care

Multiple Choice

1. After death, the muscles in the body become
   (A) Warm and pulsating
   (B) Bendable
   (C) Stiff and rigid
   (D) Hot and sharp

2. Caring for a body after death is called
   (A) Postmortem care
   (B) Mortician care
   (C) Funeral home care
   (D) Before-burial care

3. After death, the nursing assistant should place drainage pads under the body. These pads are most often needed under the
   (A) Arms
   (B) Perineum
   (C) Axillary area
   (D) Feet

4. If family members would like to remain with their loved one's body after death, the nursing assistant should
   (A) Let them do so
   (B) Inform them that the NA needs to ask the doctor first
   (C) Ask them to perform the postmortem care since they are staying with the body
   (D) Talk to them about the importance of organ donation

10. Understand and respect different postmortem practices

True or False

1. ____ Most people grieve in the same way.

2. ____ Some people like to remain with the body to perform religious rituals.

3. ____ The overall mood at a wake is usually very sad and somber.

4. ____ Having an open casket means the preserved body will be displayed to others.

5. ____ Some people will choose to be cremated, which means the body is burned until it is reduced to ashes.

6. ____ Readings of religious scripture and prayers may take place at a funeral.

7. ____ An atheist's funeral will normally involve prayers, hymns, and other religious rituals.

8. ____ The nursing assistant should remain professional and respectful whether or not he agrees with the rituals that take place after a resident has died.

9. ____ With a natural burial, the body is embalmed before placing it directly into the ground.

24

Introduction to Home Care

1. Explain the purpose of and need for home health care

Fill in the Blank

1. Home care is less

   _____

   than a long hospital or extended care facility stay.

2. The growing numbers of

   _____

   people and

   _____

   people are also creating a demand for home care services.

3. One of the most important reasons for health care in the home is that most people who are ill or disabled feel more comfortable at _____.

2. Describe a typical home health agency

Labeling
Fill in the four blanks below to complete the organizational chart of a typical home health agency.

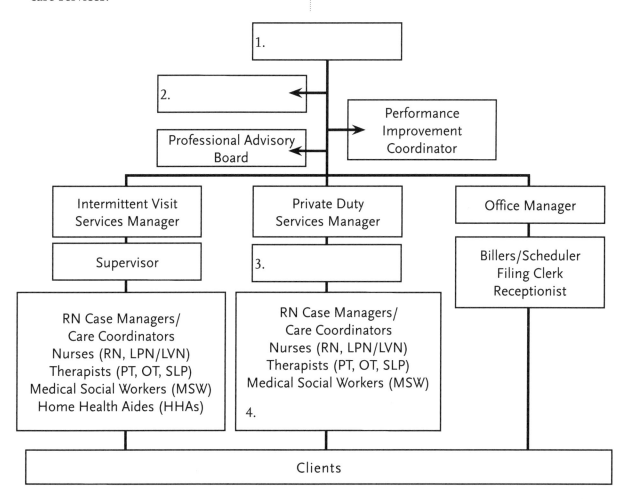

3. Explain how working for a home health agency is different from working in other types of facilities

Fill in the Blank

1. Home health aides (HHAs) must be aware of personal

   _____

   when traveling to visit clients.

2. HHAs may have a lot more contact with clients'

   _____

   in the home than they would in a facility.

3. A supervisor monitors an HHA's work, but the HHA will spend most of his hours working with clients without direct supervision. Thus, he must be independent and

   _____.

4. Careful written and verbal

   _____

   skills are important.

5. HHAs need to be

   _____

   in order to adapt to the changes in the environment.

6. In a client's home, the HHA is a

   _____

   and should be respectful of the client's property and customs.

4. Discuss the client care plan and explain how team members contribute to the care plan

True or False

1. _____ The purpose of the client care plan is to give suggestions for care, which the home health aide can customize for each client.

2. _____ Home health aides should not perform activities that are not listed on the care plan.

Short Answer

List contributions that each of the following care team members might make in developing the care plan.

3. Home Health Aide (HHA)

   _____

   _____

   _____

   _____

   _____

4. Case Manager or Supervisor

   _____

   _____

   _____

   _____

   _____

   _____

5. Physician (MD or DO)

   _____

   _____

   _____

   _____

   _____

6. Medical Social Worker (MSW)

   _____

   _____

   _____

   _____

   _____

5. Describe the role of the home health aide and explain typical tasks performed

Short Answer

1. List and give examples of two ways in which home health aides provide services to their clients.

    _____

    _____

    _____

    _____

True or False

2. _____ Home health aides never administer medications unless they are trained and assigned to do so.

3. _____ Home health aides are trained to perform invasive procedures.

4. _____ Home health aides should ignore any requests that are outside their scope of practice.

5. _____ Home health aides must not accept any request that is not part of their job description or that is not on the assignment sheet.

6. _____ The correct way to deal with unacceptable requests is to explain why the request cannot be met and report it to the supervisor.

7. _____ Home health aides should not perform procedures that require sterile technique.

8. _____ It is acceptable for home health aides to prescribe certain medications if they have permission from their supervisor.

9. _____ Home health aides should only inform the client or family of the diagnosis or medical treatment plan if the client asks.

10. _____ Home health aides may perform any task for which they have been trained, even if it is not on their assignment sheet.

6. Explain common policies and procedures for home health aides

Short Answer

1. List five examples of common policies and procedures at home health agencies.

    _____

    _____

    _____

    _____

    _____

    _____

    _____

    _____

7. Demonstrate how to organize care assignments

Short Answer

1. Why it is important for a home health aide to organize his work?

    _____

    _____

    _____

    _____

    _____

2. Why should the home health aide include the client in planning her schedule?

    _____

    _____

    _____

    _____

    _____

    _____

8. Identify an employer's responsibilities

Short Answer

List and describe four responsibilities of the employer to the home health aide.

1. _____

   _____

2. _____

   _____

3. _____

   _____

4. _____

9. Identify the client's rights in home health care

True or False

1. _____ If a home health aide suspects that a client is being abused, he should keep quiet until he gathers proof that the abuse is actually happening.

2. _____ Clients have the legal right to participate in their care planning.

3. _____ Clients should only be informed of obstacles or barriers to their care if they are life-threatening.

4. _____ Clients do not need to know what they are being charged for, as long as they are receiving adequate care.

5. _____ Home health agencies must give clients a list of their rights and review each right with them.

25

Infection Prevention and Safety in the Home

1. Discuss disinfection in the home

Short Answer

1. How does wet heat disinfect? How does dry heat disinfect?

_____

_____

_____

_____

_____

_____

_____

_____

_____

_____

2. What is the difference between sterilization and disinfection?

_____

_____

_____

_____

_____

_____

_____

_____

_____

2. Describe guidelines for assisting a client when isolation has been ordered

Multiple Choice

1. Which of the following statements is true of Transmission-Based Precautions?
   (A) Transmission-Based Precautions are used instead of Standard Precautions for clients who have an infectious disease.
   (B) Transmission-Based Precautions are used in addition to Standard Precautions for clients who have an infectious disease.
   (C) Transmission-Based Precautions are used for clients who are combative or are at risk of hurting themselves.
   (D) Transmission-Based Precautions are only used in long-term care facilities, not in the home.

2. How should a home health aide (HHA) wash the dishes when a client has an infectious disease?
   (A) The HHA should wash dishes in cold water with lemon juice.
   (B) The HHA should clean dishes with a scrubbing brush and lukewarm water.
   (C) The HHA should wash dishes in hot water with antibacterial soap.
   (D) The HHA should hold dishes over a pan of boiling water for several minutes.

3. What chemical solution can be mixed with water to disinfect contaminated surfaces?
   (A) Bleach
   (B) Corn starch
   (C) Juice
   (D) Salt

4. When collecting soiled laundry from a client's bedroom, where should the HHA bag the laundry before it is taken to be washed?
   (A) Laundry area
   (B) Empty room
   (C) Kitchen
   (D) Client's bedroom

5. What type of equipment should be limited when working with a client who has an infectious disease?
   (A) Non-disposable equipment
   (B) Blood pressure equipment
   (C) Disposable equipment
   (D) New equipment

Scenario
Read the following scenario and answer the questions below.

Eddie, a home health aide, takes a urine sample from his client, Mr. Velasquez. When Eddie finishes, he accidentally knocks the container onto the linoleum floor. Some of the urine spills onto the floor. Eddie quickly grabs a sponge and begins to wipe up the spill. When he is finished, he finds the mop, puts dishwashing soap into a bucket, and cleans the area again. When he is done mopping, he washes his hands.

6. Did Eddie follow the proper spill-handling procedure? If not, what should Eddie have done?

   _____

   _____

   _____

   _____

   _____

   _____

   _____

   _____

   _____

   _____

3. List ways to adapt the home to principles of proper body mechanics

Multiple Choice

1. If a home health aide (HHA) cannot reach an object on a high shelf, she should
   (A) Stand on tiptoes to reach it
   (B) Use a step stool
   (C) Climb on a counter
   (D) Use an umbrella to reach it

2. When sitting for long periods of time, legs should not be crossed because
   (A) It disrupts the alignment of the body
   (B) It can wrinkle a person's clothing
   (C) It is unprofessional
   (D) HHAs must stand while working

3. To be more comfortable doing tasks that require standing for long periods of time, an HHA can
   (A) Sit down every five minutes
   (B) Hop on one foot
   (C) Jump up and down
   (D) Place one foot on a footrest

4. Frequently used tools and supplies should be placed
   (A) On shelves or counters to reduce the need for bending
   (B) On the floor to reduce the need for straining to reach
   (C) In boxes where they will be out of the way
   (D) In the attic

5. To clean a bathtub, an HHA should
   (A) Bend over
   (B) Sit down on the floor
   (C) Kneel or use a low stool
   (D) Sit inside the tub

4. Identify common types of accidents in the home and describe prevention guidelines

Labeling
In the following illustrations, circle everything you can find that is unsafe.

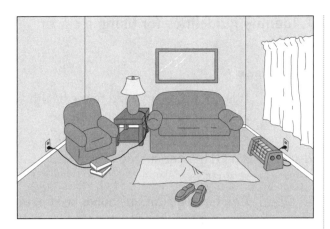

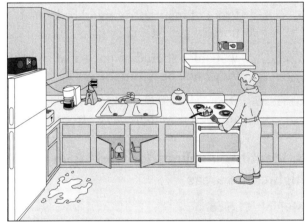

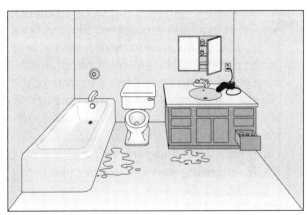

True or False

1. _____ Adjustable beds should be raised to their highest position each time the home health aide has finished with care.

2. _____ Older people are often more seriously injured by falls because their bones are more fragile.

3. _____ Older adults or people with loss of sensation due to paralysis or diabetes are at the greatest risk of burns.

4. _____ Clients should be sitting down before hot drinks are served to help prevent scalds.

5. _____ Infants should sleep on their backs to prevent sudden infant death syndrome (SIDS).

6. _____ To avoid choking, clients should eat in a reclined position.

7. _____ To promote safety in the kitchen, pot handles should be turned out of sight and toward the back of the stove.

8. _____ A client who is ill and weak should not be left alone in a tub.

5. List home fire hazards and describe fire safety guidelines

Short Answer

1. List four things that could be fire hazards.

   _____

   _____

   _____

   _____

   _____

   _____

2. What is important to remember about clothing while working near the stove?

   _____

   _____

   _____

   _____

   _____

3. How often should the smoke alarm be checked?

   _____

   _____

   _____

6. Identify ways to reduce the risk of automobile accidents

Multiple Choice

1. When driving to a new client's house, a home health aide should
   (A) Study the map while driving there
   (B) Plan the route before leaving
   (C) Call the client to discuss the day's assignments beforehand
   (D) Text a friend for directions

2. While driving, it is a good idea for the HHA to
   (A) Keep her eyes on the road and her hands on the wheel
   (B) Call her friends to pass the time more quickly
   (C) Drive quickly so she will have more time at the client's home
   (D) Send text messages to confirm the day's schedule

3. When backing up in a car, the HHA should
   (A) Only use the rearview mirror or camera
   (B) Back up quickly
   (C) Check the rearview mirror or camera and turn her head to look behind her
   (D) Use her instincts to tell if someone is behind her

4. Driving at a safe speed means
   (A) Exceeding the speed limit
   (B) Making adjustments for road or weather conditions
   (C) Driving faster if it is snowing
   (D) Going ten miles per hour under the speed limit

5. Seat belts should always be worn because
   (A) They prevent accidents
   (B) They help protect a person if an accident occurs
   (C) They make the person look more professional
   (D) They make it safer to drive much faster

7. Identify guidelines for using a car on the job

True or False

1. ____ It is not necessary for a home health aide to keep track of the miles he drives for work.

2. ____ An HHA's car should be serviced regularly.

3. ____ Proof of registration should be kept in the car at all times.

4. ____ Proof of insurance should be kept at home where it will be safe.

5. ____ Valuables should be put out of sight if they must be left in the car.

6. ____ Doors should be locked while driving and before walking away from the car.

8. Identify guidelines for working in high-crime areas

Multiple Choice

1. A home health aide is going to visit a client who lives in a high-crime area. She has been to this client's apartment before, but today as she drives up, she notices three strange men standing on the sidewalk in front of the client's apartment. They are watching her as she slows down in front of the client's apartment. What should the HHA do?
   (A) Ignore them and park the car
   (B) Keep driving past and use her phone to call her supervisor
   (C) Stop and ask them what they are doing in front of the client's apartment
   (D) Ask them to help her move items from her trunk into the client's house

2. A home health aide is getting ready to leave a client's home as it begins to get dark. Her client lives in a large house on a street that is not well-lit. She has parked next to the nearest street light, which is two houses down. What should she do on her way to her car?
   (A) Run to the car
   (B) Keep her keys inside her purse
   (C) Hold her purse or bag away from her body
   (D) Walk purposefully and confidently

26

Medications in Home Care

1. List four guidelines for safe and proper use of medications

True or False

1. _____ Home health aides must not handle or give medications unless specifically trained and assigned to do so.

2. _____ Home health aides are not allowed to touch the client's medication containers in any way.

3. _____ It is not important for the home health aide to know what medications the client is taking, as long as the HHA documents when they are taken.

4. _____ Home health aides should report symptoms such as stomachache or vomiting because these could indicate a side effect or drug interaction.

5. _____ Aspirin and ibuprofen are examples of over-the-counter drugs.

2. Identify the five "rights" of medications

Multiple Choice

1. Checking the label for instructions on how the medication should be taken is which right of medication?
   (A) The Right Client
   (B) The Right Route
   (C) The Right Time
   (D) The Right Medication

2. Checking the label for instructions on how much medication to take is which right of medication?
   (A) The Right Amount
   (B) The Right Client
   (C) The Right Time
   (D) The Right Route

3. Making sure the medication name on the container matches the name listed in the care plan is which right of medication?
   (A) The Right Time
   (B) The Right Medication
   (C) The Right Client
   (D) The Right Amount

4. Checking the label to make sure the client's name is on it is which right of medication?
   (A) The Right Client
   (B) The Right Medication
   (C) The Right Time
   (D) The Right Route

5. Checking the label for instructions on how often the medication should be taken is which right of medication?
   (A) The Right Route
   (B) The Right Client
   (C) The Right Time
   (D) The Right Amount

3. Explain how to assist a client with self-administered medications

True or False

1. _____ All medications should be taken with food to avoid stomach irritation.

Name: _____

2. ____ To avoid any problems with drug interactions, the home health aide should document every medication the client takes, whether it is part of the treatment plan or not.

3. ____ Sedatives should never be mixed with alcohol.

4. ____ The home health aide can remind a client when it is time to take medication.

5. ____ Allergic reactions to medication may require emergency help.

Short Answer

6. List seven ways in which home health aides may help clients with self-medication.

_____

_____

_____

_____

_____

_____

_____

_____

_____

_____

7. List ten things involving self-medication that home health aides are NOT allowed to do.

_____

_____

_____

_____

_____

_____

_____

_____

_____

_____

_____

_____

8. Name five common side effects that clients may experience from their medications.

_____

_____

_____

_____

_____

4. Identify observations about medications that should be reported right away

Short Answer

1. What should the home health aide do if a client shows signs of a reaction to a medication or complains of side effects?

_____

_____

_____

2. What should the home health aide do if a client takes medication in the wrong amount, at the wrong time, or takes the wrong kind of medication?

_____

_____

_____

5. Describe what to do in an emergency involving medications

Short Answer

1. Ms. Roslin takes several prescription medications each day as ordered by her physician. On the day her home health aide (HHA) is scheduled to visit her, the HHA arrives at

Ms. Roslin's home to find her sitting down in a chair and looking very ill. When the HHA asks her if she is okay, Ms. Roslin says that she feels very sick to her stomach and she thinks she might faint. Ms. Roslin says that she might have taken too much medication because she could not remember if she had already taken her morning dosage. What would be the best response by the HHA?

_____

_____

_____

_____

_____

_____

_____

_____

2. The home health aide arrives at Mr. Adama's home at 8:30 a.m. and finds him lying in bed. The HHA is unable to wake him, and then notices several bottles of pills on the table next to the bed. They are all open, and some of the pills are scattered on the table and the floor. What would be the best response by the HHA?

_____

_____

_____

_____

_____

_____

_____

_____

_____

_____

_____

6. Identify methods of medication storage

True or False

1. ____ The client's medication should be kept separate from medicine used by other members of the household.

2. ____ If young children are present in the home, medications should be stored on top of the counter.

3. ____ Medications should be stored away from heat and light.

4. ____ If medication has expired, the home health aide should discard it in the trash.

7. Identify signs of drug misuse and abuse and know how to report these

Multiple Choice

1. Proper medication use includes which of the following?
    (A) Refusing to take medications
    (B) Taking medication with alcohol
    (C) Sharing medication with others
    (D) Taking the right dose at the right time

2. The best thing the home health aide can do if a client refuses to take medication is to
    (A) Push the client to take the medication, explaining that it is good for him
    (B) Try to find out why the client does not want to take the medication, and report to the supervisor
    (C) Call 911 for emergency medical help
    (D) Call the client's doctor immediately

3. A common reason why people avoid taking prescribed medication is
    (A) They dislike the side effects
    (B) They are stubborn
    (C) They do not want to feel better
    (D) They would rather get well without it

4. Signs of drug misuse or abuse include
    (A) Increased appetite and weight gain
    (B) Unusual cheerfulness
    (C) Depression and moodiness
    (D) Better relationships with family members

Name: _____

5. The drugs that pose the highest risk for causing drug dependency are
    (A) Pain medications
    (B) Antihistamines (allergy medicines)
    (C) Beta blockers
    (D) Multivitamins

27

New Mothers, Infants, and Children

1. Explain the growth of home care for new mothers and infants

True or False

1. _____ Most new mothers stay in the hospital for several days to a week after childbirth.

2. _____ Bed rest is ordered if a woman shows signs of early labor.

3. _____ A home health aide may be needed when an expectant mother is put on bed rest by her doctor.

4. _____ New mothers today are generally more energetic when they come home than women in the past.

5. _____ Bed rest may help prevent labor from starting before the baby is ready to be born.

6. _____ Natural childbirth has been increasing in popularity.

2. Identify common neonatal disorders

Short Answer

1. List three common neonatal disorders.

_____

_____

_____

_____

_____

_____

3. Explain how to provide postpartum care

Fill in the Blank
Use this list of words and phrases to fill in the blanks in the following sentences.

Bathing   Lactation

Cesarean section   Lochia

Diapering   Monitor

Episiotomy   Pink

Feeding   Red

Housekeeping

1. An incision sometimes made in the perineal area during vaginal delivery to enlarge the vaginal opening for the baby's head is a(n)

_____.

2. The home health aide may need to monitor the amount and color of the new mother's

_____,

which is the vaginal flow that occurs after giving birth.

3. Basic care for the baby includes

_____,

_____,

and _____.

4. The home health aide may be required to do light _____ to help the new mother.

5. A surgical procedure in which the baby is delivered through an incision in the mother's abdomen is called a

_____.

6. Home health aides may be asked to

_____

the equipment if the baby is receiving oxygen.

Name: _____

7.   During the first several days, the color of lochia usually changes from bright _____ to _____.

8.   If a new mother needs help with breastfeeding, a _____ consultant can help.

4. List important observations to report and document

Short Answer

Read this scenario and answer the questions that follow.

The home health aide (HHA) arrives at a client's house at 8 a.m. to care for baby Eric, a two-day-old newborn, and finds the house dirty, the new mother Anne in a sitz bath, and baby Eric in the crib crying. The mother is also crying and complains of getting "no sleep last night." What course of action should the HHA take? How would the HHA document this?

_____
_____
_____
_____
_____
_____
_____
_____
_____
_____
_____
_____
_____
_____
_____
_____
_____

5. Explain guidelines for safely handling a baby

Labeling

Label the type of hold shown in each photo.

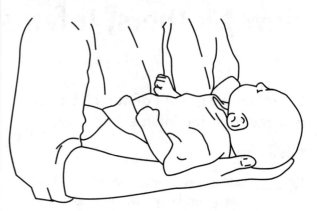

1. _____

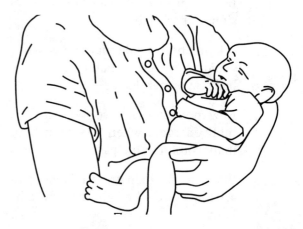

2. _____

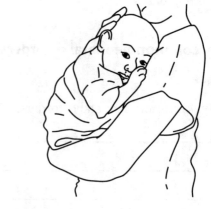

3. _____

6. Describe guidelines for assisting with feeding a baby

Multiple Choice

1. If the baby does not latch onto the nipple right away, the mother should stroke his
    (A) Toes
    (B) Elbows
    (C) Cheek
    (D) Forehead

2. Many professionals recommend that mothers try breastfeeding for _____ week(s) before deciding whether to continue or stop.
    (A) Five
    (B) Ten
    (C) One
    (D) Two

3. Powdered formula is sold in
    (A) Crates
    (B) Cans
    (C) Sterilized pitchers
    (D) Covered plastic bowls

4. The cheapest formula is usually
    (A) Ready-to-use
    (B) Concentrated liquid
    (C) Powdered
    (D) Prepared

5. A good position for breastfeeding is
    (A) Lying face down on the bed
    (B) Sitting upright in a comfortable chair
    (C) Rocking rapidly in a chair
    (D) Bending over the crib

6. Before feeding, the home health aide should check the temperature of the formula on her wrist. It should feel
    (A) Warm
    (B) Hot
    (C) Cold
    (D) Boiling

7. The mother can break the suction of a nursing baby by
    (A) Pulling down on the baby's ears
    (B) Putting her finger in the baby's mouth
    (C) Sucking on the baby's toes
    (D) Shaking the baby

8. Which of the following is best for bottle-fed newborns?
    (A) Whole milk
    (B) Infant formula
    (C) Fruit smoothies
    (D) Skim milk

7. Explain guidelines for bathing and changing a baby

True or False

1. _____ The home health aide should wear disposable gloves when changing or bathing a baby.

2. _____ Leaving a diaper off for a few minutes when changing the baby can help prevent diaper rash.

3. _____ The proper way to test a baby's bath temperature is by dipping the baby's hand in it.

4. _____ Moisture contributes to diaper rash.

5. _____ It is okay for the home health aide to take both hands off the baby if it is for less than a minute.

6. _____ Children generally wear diapers until they are eight to 12 months old.

7. _____ Newborns will need between eight and 12 diaper changes in 24 hours.

8. _____ The home health aide should always apply baby powder after giving a baby a bath.

9. _____ It is a sign of a medical problem if a newborn baby has a loose bowel movement with every feeding.

10. _____ Babies should be changed frequently to avoid diaper rash.

8. Identify how to measure weight and length of a baby

Multiple Choice

1. When weighing a baby, the home health aide should
   (A) Keep one hand on the baby at all times
   (B) Step back from the scale after the baby is on it
   (C) Place the scale on the floor to see if the baby will crawl onto it
   (D) Stand the baby up on the scale for an accurate weight

2. How can a baby's length be determined?
   (A) By standing the baby up against a wall, making a pencil mark at the top of his head, and measuring the height of the mark
   (B) By holding the baby against the home health aide's leg and measuring how high the baby's head reaches
   (C) By placing the baby on paper, making pencil marks at the head and heel, and measuring the distance between the marks
   (D) By putting the baby on a standing scale and lowering the measuring rod until it rests flat on the baby's head

9. Explain guidelines for special care

Matching
Use each letter only once.

1. _____ Apnea

2. _____ Circumcision

3. _____ Oxygen

4. _____ Umbilical cord

(A) The cord that connects the baby to the placenta

(B) The removal of part of the foreskin of the penis

(C) The state of not breathing

(D) Given to some babies who have breathing problems; considered a medication

10. Identify special needs of children and describe how children respond to stress

Short Answer

1. List some examples of physical needs that children have.

_____

_____

_____

_____

_____

2. List one example of a mental need that children have.

_____

_____

_____

3. List four examples of emotional needs that children have.

_____

_____

_____

_____

_____

_____

4. List five reasons that children may experience stress.

_____

_____

_____

_____

_____

_____

_____

_____

5. List five factors that influence the way children respond to stress.

_____

_____

_____

_____

_____

_____

_____

_____

6. In what ways might school-age children react to stress?

_____

_____

_____

_____

_____

_____

_____

7. In what negative ways might adolescents react to stress?

_____

_____

_____

_____

_____

_____

_____

11. List symptoms of common childhood illnesses and the required care

Fill in the Blank

1. _____, cleaning, and disinfection are the best ways to prevent infection.

2. Frequent loose or watery bowel movements are called _____.

3. Children with diarrhea may experience

   _____,

   thus doctors may recommend electrolyte replacement drinks.

4. In general, children should not be given

   _____,

   because it has been associated with some serious disorders.

5. Treatment of a fever includes a lukewarm bath or _____.

6. When children have diarrhea, doctors usually recommend that they resume their normal, well-balanced diet within _____ hours of getting sick.

7. Rest and _____ are recommended for fevers.

8. Too much acetaminophen can cause _____ damage.

12. Identify guidelines for working with children

Scenarios
Read the following scenarios and decide how to respond.

1. Zack and his older brother Lee have just returned home from school. Zack is upset because he did not win a prize for his science project, but his brother did. He cried at school, and some of the other kids made fun of him. He becomes visibly distressed again as he relates this story to the home health aide at his home. What would be the best response by the home health aide?

_____

_____

Name: _____

_____

_____

_____

_____

_____

_____

_____

2. The home health aide notices that Kara has been withdrawn all afternoon. She did not go outside to play after school, and at dinner she refuses to eat anything. She makes comments like "nobody cares about me." What would be the best response by the home health aide?

_____

_____

_____

_____

_____

_____

_____

_____

_____

_____

_____

13. List the signs of child abuse and neglect and know how to report them

Short Answer

1. Psychological abuse of children includes

_____

_____

_____

_____

_____

_____

2. Sexual abuse of children includes

_____

_____

_____

_____

_____

_____

3. Child neglect is

_____

_____

_____

_____

28

Meal Planning, Shopping, Preparation, and Storage

1. Explain how to prepare a basic food plan and list food shopping guidelines

Short Answer
Make a basic food plan for Monday through Friday. Include breakfast, lunch, dinner, and snacks.

MONDAY

Breakfast

Snack

Lunch

Snack

Dinner

Snack

TUESDAY

Breakfast

Snack

Lunch

Snack

Dinner

Snack

WEDNESDAY

Breakfast

Snack

Lunch

Snack

Dinner

Snack

THURSDAY

Breakfast

Snack

Lunch

Snack

Dinner

Snack

Name: _____

_____

_____

_____

_____

_____

FRIDAY
_____

Breakfast

Snack

Lunch

Snack

Dinner

Snack
_____

Fill in the Blank

1. Avoid _____,
   already-mixed, or ready-made foods because
   they are more expensive.

2. Read _____
   for ingredients that may be harmful to the
   client, such as excessive salt.

3. Estimate the _____
   by dividing the total cost by the number of
   servings.

4. For clients on a low-fat diet, take the
   _____
   off chicken and turkey parts.

5. Buy fresh foods that are in season when they
   are at their _____
   flavor.

6. Large amounts or larger sizes are usually
   more _____.

7. Cheaper cuts of meat tend to have more
   _____
   in bones and fat.

Short Answer

8. List four factors that the home health aide
   should consider when buying food.

   _____

   _____

   _____

2. List and define common health claims on food labels

Fill in the Blank

1. _____ meat,
   poultry, eggs, and dairy products come from
   animals that are given no antibiotics or
   growth hormones.

2. _____
   products may contain artificial sweeteners,
   such as saccharin or aspartame.

3. If a product is labeled
   _____ or
   _____, it
   usually does not contain much fat.

4. The claims of
   _____,
   healthy, or *good for you* may have little or no
   meaning.

5. Clients who must reduce their sodium or
   salt intake should eat foods labeled
   _____,
   _____, or
   _____.

6. The best way to limit
   _____
   is to avoid foods containing animal fats.

7. If a product is labeled
   _____, it
   means that the chickens producing the eggs
   have been allowed access to the outside for
   an unspecified period of time.

3. Explain the information on the FDA-required Nutrition Facts label

Multiple Choice

1. In the updated version of the label, a new subcategory was added called:
   (A) Added carbohydrates
   (B) Added minerals
   (C) Added proteins
   (D) Added sugars

2. Which of the following minerals is required to be on the nutrition facts label?
   (A) Zinc
   (B) Selenium
   (C) Phosphate
   (D) Iron

3. The standardized nutrition label on all packaged foods is called
   (A) Percentage label
   (B) Food Information label
   (C) Nutrition Facts label
   (D) Serving Size Information label

4. The recommended daily totals on the label are based on a _____-calorie diet.
   (A) 2,500
   (B) 2,000
   (C) 1,000
   (D) 5,000

4. List guidelines for safe food preparation

True or False

1. _____ The home health aide (HHA) should wash his hands before handling food, but does not need to wash his hands again afterward.

2. _____ Sponges can be washed in the dishwasher to disinfect them.

3. _____ It is a good idea to defrost frozen foods on the counter.

4. _____ Refrigerated food can be left out on the counter safely for five hours.

5. _____ Poultry needs to be cooked thoroughly to kill microorganisms.

6. _____ If the HHA sneezes while around food, she should wash her hands again.

7. _____ It is best to use separate cutting boards for meat and vegetables.

8. _____ It is not necessary to change knives between cutting fresh meat and vegetables.

9. _____ If a person has a weakened immune system because of cancer, a foodborne illness can be deadly.

10. _____ Elderly people are at increased risk for foodborne illnesses because they do not care about how food tastes.

5. Identify methods of food preparation

Matching
For each method of food preparation, identify the correct description. Use each letter only once.

1. _____ Baking

2. _____ Boiling

3. _____ Braising

4. _____ Broiling

5. _____ Frying

6. _____ Microwaving

7. _____ Poaching

8. _____ Roasting

9. _____ Sautéing

10. _____ Steaming

(A) Safe for defrosting, reheating, and cooking, but this method can cause cold spots.

(B) Cooked in barely boiling water or other liquids; this is an ideal way to prepare fish and eggs.

(C) Used for meats, poultry, and some vegetables, this method may involve mixing items with oils or spices before cooking, and basting meats or poultry during cooking.

(D) The best method for cooking pasta, noodles, and rice.

(E) Used in an oven at a moderate heat, this method is appropriate for many foods such as breads, fish, vegetables, and casseroles.

(F) A quick way to cook vegetables and meats by using a small amount of oil in a frying pan and stirring constantly.

(G) A small amount of water is boiled in the bottom of a saucepan, and food is set over it in a basket or colander.

(H) The least healthy way to cook, this method uses a lot of fat.

(I) This method can be used to melt cheese or brown the top of a casserole.

(J) A slow-cooking method that uses moist heat to cook meat or vegetables at a temperature just below boiling.

6. Identify four methods of low-fat food preparation

Fill in the Blank

1. _____ allows fats in meat to drip out before food is consumed, which lowers fat content.

2. Plan meals around _____ to help cut out the fat content.

3. Sometimes high-fat ingredients can be _____ or replaced to lower the fat content of a recipe.

4. _____ meat on paper towels after browning it.

5. Leave out _____ on sandwiches or on tops of casseroles.

6. An example of a low-fat meal based on grains is beans and _____.

7. Boiling, steaming, broiling, roasting, and _____ are all methods of cooking that require little fat.

8. Try substituting regular or Greek _____ for mayonnaise or sour cream.

7. List four guidelines for safe food storage

Multiple Choice

1. After shopping, which of the following foods should be put away first?
   (A) Crackers
   (B) Milk
   (C) Pasta
   (D) Cereal

2. It is a good idea to keep easily spoiled items in the
   (A) Door of the refrigerator
   (B) Cupboard
   (C) Rear of the refrigerator
   (D) Pantry

3. Refrigerator temperature should be
   (A) 0°F–10°F
   (B) 36°F–40°F
   (C) 10°F–20°F
   (D) 62°F–66°F

4. Food can be safely left out for _____ hours.
   (A) Five
   (B) Three
   (C) Two
   (D) Twelve

5. If the home health aide is not sure whether food is spoiled, she should
   (A) Discard it
   (B) Cook it at a higher heat than usual
   (C) Cook it for a longer time than usual
   (D) Smell it after cooking it to be sure it is okay

6. Foods that can be composted include
   (A) Canola oil
   (B) Fish bones
   (C) Yogurt
   (D) Coffee grounds

29

The Clean, Safe, and Healthy Home Environment

1. Describe how housekeeping affects physical and psychological well-being

Short Answer

1. What are some of the reasons that home health aides should maintain an orderly and clean household for their clients?

_____
_____
_____
_____
_____
_____
_____
_____
_____
_____
_____
_____

2. List qualities needed to manage a home and describe general housekeeping guidelines

True or False

1. _____ The home health aide's (HHA) primary responsibility is to clean the client's kitchen.

2. _____ The HHA should expect that all members of the household will be able to help with housekeeping.

3. _____ One HHA assignment might be managing a client's finances.

4. _____ The HHA will need to be flexible with regard to household maintenance.

5. _____ Vacuuming is not part of an HHA's duties.

6. _____ Using proper body mechanics when performing housekeeping activities helps prevent injury.

7. _____ It is important for HHAs to be sensitive to each client's customs and beliefs.

8. _____ The HHA will need to use cleaning materials and methods that are approved by clients and their families.

9. _____ The HHA should clean up and straighten up after every activity.

10. _____ One HHA responsibility is observing for infestation of insects and animals.

3. Describe cleaning products and equipment

True or False

1. _____ All-purpose cleaners can be used on several types of surfaces.

2. _____ For really dirty surfaces, it is best to use a mixture of bleach and ammonia.

3. _____ Abrasive cleaners are used mostly for bathing clients.

4. _____ A sponge is generally used to soften and remove soil on washable surfaces.

5. _____ Vacuum cleaner bags should be checked frequently.

6. ____ Some cleaning products can cause burns.

7. ____ Lemon juice is an example of an environmentally-friendly cleaning solution.

8. ____ White vinegar mixed with water can be used to clean glass.

9. ____ Baking soda is a type of toxic abrasive scouring powder.

4. Describe proper cleaning methods for living areas, kitchens, bathrooms, and storage areas

Multiple Choice

1. Examples of essential items that should be kept within reach of the client include
   (A) Eyeglasses
   (B) Potato chips
   (C) Nail polish
   (D) Cosmetics

2. Falls and accidents in the home are often caused by
   (A) Well-lit hallways
   (B) Wet floors
   (C) Clean floors
   (D) Leftover food scraps

3. In the kitchen, diseases may be transmitted by
   (A) Soap
   (B) Medications
   (C) Contaminated food surfaces
   (D) Bleach

4. It is a good idea for the home health aide to dust this frequently, unless the client has allergies:
   (A) Five times a week
   (B) Once a week
   (C) Once every two months
   (D) Twice a month

5. If the freezer is not self-defrosting, the home health aide can quickly defrost it by
   (A) Using a warm knife to chip at the ice
   (B Lighting matches near the ice
   (C) Holding a lighter near the ice
   (D) Placing pans of hot water in it

6. In order to remove odors, the home health aide can use
   (A) Flour
   (B) Baking soda
   (C) Sugar
   (D) Baking powder

7. Dishes can be sterilized by
   (A) Using a dishwasher
   (B) Using cold water
   (C) Using an oven cleaner
   (D) Drying them with a dish towel

8. How often should the home health aide dispose of garbage?
   (A) Daily
   (B) Weekly
   (C) Monthly
   (D) Every two weeks

9. Basic bathroom hygiene includes
   (A) Washing from dirty areas to clean areas
   (B) Placing soiled towels on the bathroom sink
   (C) Cleaning the tub and shower after each use
   (D) Leaving toothbrushes in the sink

10. Instead of glass cleaner, the home health aide can mix water and ____ to clean glass.
    (A) White wine
    (B) White vinegar
    (C) Apple juice
    (D) Spray starch

11. In what situation do mold and mildew grow best?
    (A) In extreme cold
    (B) In dry heat
    (C) In warm, moist places
    (D) In windy areas

12. Floors and rugs should be vacuumed at least
    (A) Once a month
    (B) Twice a week
    (C) Once a week
    (D) Once a day

13. Which of the following materials is commonly recycled?
    (A) Wood
    (B) Plastic
    (C) Polyester
    (D) Marble

5. Describe how to prepare a cleaning schedule

Create a sample cleaning schedule for an immobile client.

Immediately:

_____

_____

_____

_____

_____

Daily:

_____

_____

_____

_____

_____

Weekly:

_____

_____

_____

_____

_____

Monthly:

_____

_____

_____

_____

_____

Less often:

_____

_____

_____

_____

_____

6. List special housekeeping procedures to use when infection is present

Fill in the Blank

1. _____
   any surfaces that come into contact with body fluids, such as
   _____,
   urinals, and toilets.

2. Frequently remove
   _____ containing
   used tissues.

3. Keep any _____
   of urine, stool, or sputum in double bags away from food.

4. Take special _____
   in housecleaning when the client has an infectious disease.

5. _____ dishes and
   utensils should be used for the client.

6. Wash dishes in hot, soapy water with
   _____, and rinse
   in _____ water.

7. _____ the client's
   bathroom daily.

Name: _____

7. Explain how to do laundry and care for clothes

Crossword

Across

2. What bleach must always be diluted with

5. Washing cycle used for delicate or fragile items

6. Washing cycle used for sturdy permanent press items and cottons

8. Type of bleach used on washable fabrics; most effective in hot water

9. Delicate fabric requires _____ time in the dryer.

10. If clients can do their own mending, the HHA may just need to _____ the needle.

11. Water temperature used for brightly-colored fabrics

13. One way to reduce these is to fold clothes immediately after they are dried

Down

1. Water temperature used for whites and towels

2. Liquid chlorine bleach does this to clothing in addition to removing stains

3. The safest water temperature for most garments

4. If dirty or stained laundry items were specially treated before washing, they were

_____.

7. Must be cleaned every time the dryer is used

11. Parts of a shirt that should be ironed first, after collars

12. Pressing dark fabrics and silks on the wrong side helps prevent them from looking like this

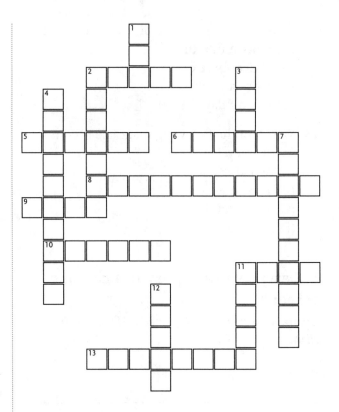

8. List special laundry precautions to take when infection is present

True or False

1. ____ It is best to use cold water when doing laundry for a client who has an infectious disease.

2. ____ The home health aide should wear gloves when doing an infectious client's laundry.

3. ____ Dirty laundry should be shaken to remove dirt before putting it in the washing machine.

4. ____ The home health aide should keep an infectious client's laundry separate from other family members' laundry.

5. ____ Dirty laundry should remain in the client's room as long as possible to avoid contamination of the rest of the house.

6. ____ Agency-approved disinfectants should be used in loads of laundry.

9. List guidelines for teaching housekeeping skills to clients' family members

Scenario

Read the following scenario and decide how to respond.

1. Dave, a home health aide, is explaining to Mrs. Crawford's family how to protect against infectious diseases when doing the laundry and cleaning the kitchen. He has written a long list of instructions, and when he has finished explaining, two family members still seem confused about some key points. How should Dave respond in this situation?

_____

_____

_____

_____

_____

_____

_____

_____

_____

_____

_____

10. Identify hazardous household materials

Short Answer

1. Identify five hazardous household materials.

_____

_____

_____

_____

_____

Name: _____

30

Managing Time, Energy, and Money in the Home

1. Explain ways to work more efficiently

Short Answer

1. For each of the ways of working more efficiently described in the guidelines in this learning objective, give an example (other than what is in the book) of how you can put the method into action.

_____

_____

_____

_____

_____

_____

_____

_____

_____

_____

_____

_____

_____

_____

2. List five ways to conserve time and energy.

_____

_____

_____

_____

_____

_____

2. Describe how to follow an established work plan with the client and family

Short Answer

1. Pick the busiest day you will have next week, and draft a work plan for that day. List tasks to complete and prioritize them.

_____

_____

_____

_____

_____

_____

_____

_____

_____

_____

_____

_____

_____

_____

_____

_____

_____

_____

_____

_____

_____

3. Discuss ways to handle inappropriate requests

Scenario
Read the following scenario and answer the question.

1. Zoe, a home health aide, is preparing to leave her client's home for the day. Mr. Perez, her client, demands that Zoe buy him some soup at the grocery store before she leaves. This errand is not in the care plan, but Mr. Perez tells her that he really wants some soup. Mr. Perez begins to cry. What should Zoe do in this situation?

_____
_____
_____
_____
_____
_____
_____
_____
_____
_____

4. List money-saving homemaking tips

Short Answer

1. List and briefly explain five money-saving tips.

_____
_____
_____
_____
_____
_____

_____
_____
_____
_____
_____
_____

5. List guidelines for handling a client's money

Short Answer

1. What are your state's guidelines for handling a client's money?

_____
_____
_____
_____
_____
_____

True or False

2. _____ It is fine for a home health aide (HHA) to use her client's money for her own things as long as she pays it back quickly.

3. _____ It is a good idea for the HHA to estimate the amount of money he will need before requesting it.

4. _____ The HHA should return receipts to the client or family member as soon as possible.

5. _____ The HHA should keep a client's cash separate from her own.

6. _____ If a client is unsure about his budget, the HHA should give him financial advice and budgeting tips.

31

Caring for Your Career and Yourself

1. Discuss different types of careers in the healthcare field

True or False

1. _____ Direct service workers include salespeople, waiters, and bartenders.

2. _____ X-ray technicians work in diagnostic services.

3. _____ Receptionists, office managers, and billing staff are considered part of the healthcare field.

4. _____ Health educators have job opportunities within the healthcare field.

5. _____ Counselors and social workers are not part of the healthcare field.

2. Explain how to find a job and how to write a résumé

True or False

1. _____ If a potential employer asks a person for proof of his legal status in this country, it means that the employer is being discriminatory.

2. _____ Friends and relatives are the best references to use for a potential job.

3. _____ A person's résumé should fit on one page.

4. _____ A résumé should include a list of the person's educational experience.

5. _____ A résumé should include a list of a person's religious and political beliefs.

6. _____ A cover letter should emphasize the skills that would be a good match for the position a person is seeking.

3. Demonstrate completing an effective job application

Short Answer
Complete the sample job application.

Employment Application

Personal Information

Name:		Date:

Home Address:

City, State, Zip:

Email Address:

Phone:		Business Phone:

US Citizen?	If Not, Give Visa No. and Expiration Date:

Position Applying For

Title	Salary Desired:

Referred By:	Date Available:

Education

High School (Name, City, State):

Graduation Date:

Technical or Undergraduate School:

Dates Attended:	Degree Major:

References

4. Demonstrate competence in job interview techniques

Short Answer

Make a check mark (✓) next to the descriptions that are appropriate for job interviews.

1. ____ Wearing jeans

2. ____ Looking happy to be there

3. ____ Asking if it is okay to smoke during the interview

4. ____ Wearing very little jewelry

5. ____ Asking how many hours you would work

6. ____ Bringing your child with you when you cannot find a babysitter

7. ____ Wearing your nicest perfume

8. ____ Sitting up straight

9. ____ Asking what benefits the employer offers

10. ____ Shaking hands with the interviewer

11. ____ Eating a granola bar during the interview

12. ____ Asking if you got the job at the end of the interview

5. Describe a standard job description

Short Answer

1. What is a job description?

_____

_____

_____

_____

_____

2. How does a job description protect employers and employees?

_____

_____

_____

_____
_____
_____
_____
_____
_____

6. Discuss how to manage and resolve conflict

Multiple Choice

1. When is an appropriate time to discuss an issue that is causing conflict in the workplace?
   (A) When the nursing assistant (NA) decides she cannot take it anymore
   (B) When the NA is angry because something has just occurred
   (C) Right before the NA gives her notice
   (D) When the supervisor has decided on a proper time and place to discuss it

2. When trying to resolve conflict, the NA should
   (A) Interrupt the other person if the NA might forget what she is going to say
   (B) Sit back in the chair with her arms crossed over her chest
   (C) Take turns speaking
   (D) Yell at the other person if it seems like her point is not understood

3. When discussing conflict, the NA should
   (A) State how she feels when a behavior occurs
   (B) Name-call
   (C) Not look the other person in the eye
   (D) Keep the TV on to fill awkward silences

4. To resolve conflict, the NA should be prepared to
   (A) Compromise
   (B) Quit
   (C) Yell
   (D) Interrupt

7. Describe employee evaluations and discuss appropriate responses to feedback

Short Answer

Read the following and mark whether they are examples of constructive feedback or hostile criticism. Use a C for constructive and an H for hostile.

1. _____ "You are a horrible person."

2. _____ "If you weren't so slow, things might get done around here."

3. _____ "Some of your reports are incomplete; try to be more careful."

4. _____ "That was the worst bath I've ever had."

5. _____ "I'm not sure that you understood what I meant. Let me rephrase the issue."

6. _____ "Where did you learn how to clean?"

7. _____ "That was a stupid idea."

8. _____ "That procedure could have been performed in a more efficient way."

9. _____ "Try to make more of an effort to listen carefully."

10. _____ "Stop being so lazy."

8. Explain how to make job changes

Fill in the Blank

1. The nursing assistant (NA) should always give an employer _____ weeks' written notice that he will be leaving.

2. Potential future employers may talk with the NA's past _____.

3. If an NA decides to change jobs, he should be _____.

9. Discuss certification and explain the state's registry

Multiple Choice

1. The Omnibus Budget Reconciliation Act (OBRA) requires that nursing assistants complete at least ___ hours of initial training before being employed.
   (A) 30
   (B) 50
   (C) 75
   (D) 100

2. OBRA requires that nursing assistants complete _____ hours of annual continuing education.
   (A) 12
   (B) 62
   (C) 75
   (D) 19

3. After completing a training course, nursing assistants are given a(n) _____ in order to be certified to work in a particular state.
   (A) Thesis document
   (B) Residency certificate
   (C) Competency evaluation
   (D) Apprenticeship

4. Information in each state's registry of nursing assistants includes
   (A) Personal preferences for grooming
   (B) Any findings of abuse or neglect
   (C) Mortgage information
   (D) Special diet requests

5. Moving nursing assistant certification from one state to another state is called
   (A) Call-back
   (B) Free trade
   (C) Interstate agreement
   (D) Reciprocity

10. Describe continuing education

True or False

1. _____ The federal government requires 20 hours of continuing education each year.

2. _____ Treatments or regulations can change.

3. _____ States require less continuing education than the federal government.

4. _____ In-service continuing education courses help keep a nursing assistant's knowledge fresh.

11. Define *stress* and *stressors*

Short Answer

1. What are some things that make you experience stress? How do you react when you are stressed?

_____

_____

_____

_____

_____

_____

_____

_____

_____

_____

_____

_____

_____

_____

_____

12. Explain ways to manage stress

Multiple Choice

1. Stress is a _____ response.
   (A) Relaxed
   (B) Physical
   (C) Rare
   (D) Supervisory

2. When the heart beats fast in stressful situations, it can be due to an increase of the hormone
   (A) Testosterone
   (B) Estrogen
   (C) Adrenaline
   (D) Progesterone

3. A healthy lifestyle includes
   (A) Eating when a person is not hungry
   (B) Exercising regularly
   (C) Smoking a few cigarettes a week
   (D) Complaining about a job

4. Which of the following is a sign that a person is not managing stress?
   (A) Preparing meals ahead of time
   (B) Taking deep breaths and relaxing
   (C) Feeling alert and positive
   (D) Not being able to focus on work

5. Which of the following are appropriate people for a nursing assistant to turn to for help in managing stress?
   (A) Residents
   (B) Supervisors
   (C) Residents' family members
   (D) Residents' friends

6. Write out your own personal stress management plan. Be sure to include things like diet, exercise, relaxation, entertainment, etc.

_____

_____

_____

_____

_____

_____

_____

_____

_____

_____

_____

_____

_____

13. Describe a relaxation technique

Short Answer

1. Try the body scan exercise on page 502 of the textbook. Describe how you felt after the experience.

_____

_____

_____

_____

_____

_____

_____

_____

_____

_____

_____

_____

2. List six things you have done in the last month that you are happy about or proud of.

_____

_____

_____

_____

_____

_____

_____

_____

_____

14. List ways to remind yourself of the importance of the work you have chosen to do

Short Answer

1. List five things you have learned in this course that have surprised or excited you.

_____

_____

_____

_____

_____

_____

_____

_____

_____

_____

_____

_____

_____

_____

2. List two things that you are looking forward to doing when you start working as a nursing assistant or home health aide.

_____

_____

_____

_____

Caring for Your Career and Yourself

_____

_____

_____

_____

_____

_____

_____

_____

_____

_____

_____

_____

Procedure Checklists

5
Infection Prevention and Control

Washing hands (hand hygiene)			
	Procedure Steps	yes	no
1.	Turns on water at sink, keeping clothes dry and away from sink.		
2.	Wets hands and wrists thoroughly.		
3.	Applies soap to hands.		
4.	Keeps hands lower than elbows and fingertips down. Rubs hands together and lathers all surfaces of wrists, fingers, and hands, using friction for at least 20 seconds.		
5.	Cleans nails by rubbing them in palm of other hand.		
6.	Keeps hands lower than elbows and fingertips down. Without touching sink, rinses all surfaces of hands and wrists, running water from wrists to fingertips.		
7.	Uses clean, dry paper towel to dry all surfaces of hands, wrists, and fingers. Disposes of towel without touching container.		
8.	Uses clean, dry paper towel to turn off faucet, then disposes of towel without contaminating hands.		

_____   _____
Date Reviewed   Instructor Signature
_____   _____
Date Performed   Instructor Signature

Putting on (donning) and removing (doffing) gown			
	Procedure Steps	yes	no
1.	Washes hands.		
2.	Opens gown and allows it to unfold without shaking it. Places arms through each sleeve.		
3.	Fastens neck opening.		
4.	Pulls gown until it completely covers clothing. Secures gown at waist.		
5.	Puts on gloves after putting on gown.		
6.	Removes and discards gloves before removing gown. Unfastens gown at neck and waist and removes gown without touching outside of gown. Rolls dirty side in, while holding gown away from body. Discards gown and washes hands.		

_____   _____
Date Reviewed   Instructor Signature
_____   _____
Date Performed   Instructor Signature

Putting on (donning) mask and goggles			
	Procedure Steps	yes	no
1.	Washes hands.		
2.	Picks up mask by top strings or elastic strap. Does not touch mask where it touches face.		
3.	Pulls elastic strap over head or ties top strings then bottom strings.		
4.	Pinches metal strip at top of mask tightly around nose.		
5.	Puts on goggles.		
6.	Puts on gloves.		

_____   _____
Date Reviewed   Instructor Signature
_____   _____
Date Performed   Instructor Signature

Putting on (donning) gloves

	Procedure Steps	yes	no
1.	Washes hands.		
2.	If right-handed, slides one glove on left hand (reverses if left-handed).		
3.	With gloved hand, slides other hand into second glove.		
4.	Interlaces fingers to smooth out folds and create a comfortable fit.		
5.	Carefully looks for tears, holes, or spots. Replaces glove if necessary.		
6.	If wearing a gown, pulls cuffs of gloves over sleeves of gown.		

_____   _____
Date Reviewed   Instructor Signature

_____   _____
Date Performed   Instructor Signature

Removing (doffing) gloves

	Procedure Steps	yes	no
1.	Touches only the outside of one glove and grasps other glove at the palm. Pulls glove off.		
2.	With ungloved hand, slips two fingers underneath cuff of the remaining glove without touching any part of the outside.		
3.	Pulls down, turning this glove inside out and over the first glove.		
4.	Discards gloves properly.		
5.	Washes hands.		

_____   _____
Date Reviewed   Instructor Signature

_____   _____
Date Performed   Instructor Signature

Donning a full set of PPE

	Procedure Steps	yes	no
1.	Washes hands.		
2.	Dons gown properly.		
3.	Dons mask properly.		
4.	Dons goggles properly.		
5.	Dons gloves properly.		

_____   _____
Date Reviewed   Instructor Signature

_____   _____
Date Performed   Instructor Signature

Doffing a full set of PPE

	Procedure Steps	yes	no
1.	Removes and discards gloves properly.		
2.	Removes goggles properly.		
3.	Removes and discards gown properly.		
4.	Removes and discards mask properly.		
5.	Washes hands.		

_____   _____
Date Reviewed   Instructor Signature

_____   _____
Date Performed   Instructor Signature

7
Emergency Care and Disaster Preparation

Performing abdominal thrusts for the conscious person

	Procedure Steps	yes	no
1.	Stands behind person and brings arms under person's arms. Wraps arms around person's waist.		

2.	Makes a fist with one hand. Places thumb side of the fist against person's abdomen, above the navel but below the breastbone.		
3.	Grasps the fist with other hand. Pulls both hands toward self and up, quickly and forcefully.		
4.	Repeats until the object is pushed out or the person loses consciousness.		
5.	Reports and documents incident.		

_____ _____
Date Reviewed   Instructor Signature

_____ _____
Date Performed   Instructor Signature

Clearing an obstructed airway in a conscious infant

	Procedure Steps	yes	no
1.	Lays the infant face down on forearm; if sitting, rests the arm holding the infant's torso on lap or thigh. Supports infant's jaw and head with hand.		
2.	Using heel of free hand, delivers up to five back blows.		
3.	If the obstruction is not expelled, turns infant onto her back while supporting the head. Delivers up to five chest thrusts.		
4.	Repeats, alternating five back blows and five chest compressions until object is pushed out or the infant loses consciousness.		
5.	Calls 911 immediately if infant loses consciousness. Reports and documents incident.		

_____ _____
Date Reviewed   Instructor Signature

_____ _____
Date Performed   Instructor Signature

Responding to shock

	Procedure Steps	yes	no
1.	Notifies nurse immediately.		
2.	Puts on gloves and controls bleeding if bleeding occurs.		
3.	Has the person lie down on her back unless bleeding from the mouth or vomiting. Elevates the legs 8 to 12 inches unless signs of injury or fractures exist.		
4.	Checks pulse and respirations if possible.		
5.	Keeps person as calm and comfortable as possible.		
6.	Maintains normal body temperature.		
7.	Does not give person anything to eat or drink.		
8.	Reports and documents incident.		

_____ _____
Date Reviewed   Instructor Signature

_____ _____
Date Performed   Instructor Signature

Responding to a myocardial infarction

	Procedure Steps	yes	no
1.	Notifies nurse immediately.		
2.	Places person in a comfortable position. Encourages him to rest and reassures him that he will not be left alone.		
3.	Loosens clothing around the neck.		
4.	Does not give person liquids or food.		
5.	Monitors person's breathing and pulse. If breathing stops or person has no pulse, performs CPR if trained to do so.		
6.	Stays with person until help arrives.		

Name: _____

		yes	no
7.	Reports and documents incident.		

_____   _____
Date Reviewed   Instructor Signature

_____   _____
Date Performed   Instructor Signature

Controlling bleeding

	Procedure Steps	yes	no
1.	Notifies nurse immediately.		
2.	Puts on gloves.		
3.	Holds thick pad, clean cloth, or clean towel against the wound.		
4.	Presses down hard directly on the bleeding wound until help arrives. Does not decrease pressure. Puts additional pads over the first pad if blood seeps through. Does not remove the first pad.		
5.	Raises the wound above the level of the heart to slow the bleeding.		
6.	When bleeding is under control, secures the dressing to keep it in place. Checks for symptoms of shock. Stays with person until help arrives.		
7.	Removes and discards gloves. Washes hands.		
8.	Reports and documents incident.		

_____   _____
Date Reviewed   Instructor Signature

_____   _____
Date Performed   Instructor Signature

Treating burns

	Procedure Steps	yes	no
	Minor burns:		
1.	Notifies nurse immediately. Puts on gloves.		

		yes	no
2.	Uses cool, clean water to decrease the skin temperature and prevent further injury (does not use ice, ice water, ointment, salve, or grease). Dampens a clean cloth and covers burn.		
3.	Covers area with dry, clean dressing or nonadhesive bandage.		
4.	Removes and discards gloves. Washes hands.		
	Serious burns:		
1.	Removes person from the source of burn.		
2.	Notifies nurse immediately. Puts on gloves.		
3.	Checks for breathing, pulse, and severe bleeding. Begins CPR if trained and allowed to do so.		
4.	Does not use ointment, water, salve, or grease. Does not remove clothing from burned areas. Covers burn with sterile gauze or a clean sheet.		
5.	Monitors vital signs and waits for emergency medical help.		
6.	Removes and discards gloves. Washes hands.		
7.	Reports and documents incident.		

_____   _____
Date Reviewed   Instructor Signature

_____   _____
Date Performed   Instructor Signature

Responding to fainting

	Procedure Steps	yes	no
1.	Notifies nurse immediately.		
2.	Has person lie down or sit down before fainting occurs.		
3.	If person is in a sitting position, has him bend forward and place his head between his knees. If person is lying flat on his back, elevates his legs.		

		yes	no
4.	Loosens any tight clothing.		
5.	Has person stay in position for at least five minutes after symptoms disappear.		
6.	Helps person get up slowly. Continues to observe her for symptoms of fainting.		
7.	If person faints, lowers him to floor and positions him on his back. Elevates the legs 8 to 12 inches if there are no injuries, and checks for breathing.		
8.	Reports and documents incident.		

_____   _____
Date Reviewed   Instructor Signature

_____   _____
Date Performed   Instructor Signature

Responding to a nosebleed

	Procedure Steps	yes	no
1.	Notifies nurse immediately.		
2.	Elevates head of the bed or tells person to remain in sitting position. Offers tissues or a clean cloth.		
3.	Puts on gloves. Applies firm pressure on both sides of the nose, on the soft part, up near the bridge. Squeezes sides of nose with thumb and forefinger.		
4.	Applies pressure until bleeding stops.		
5.	Uses a cool cloth or ice wrapped in a cloth on bridge of nose to slow blood flow.		
6.	Removes and discards gloves. Washes hands.		
7.	Reports and documents incident.		

_____   _____
Date Reviewed   Instructor Signature

_____   _____
Date Performed   Instructor Signature

Responding to a seizure

	Procedure Steps	yes	no
1.	Notes the time and puts on gloves.		
2.	Lowers person to the floor and loosens clothing. Tries to turn person's head to one side.		
3.	Has someone call nurse immediately or uses call light. Does not leave person unless has to get medical help.		
4.	Moves furniture away to prevent injury.		
5.	Does not try to restrain the person.		
6.	Does not force anything between the person's teeth. Does not place hands in person's mouth.		
7.	Does not give liquids or food.		
8.	When the seizure is over, notes time and turns person on left side if injury is not suspected. Checks breathing and pulse. Begins CPR if breathing and pulse are absent and if trained and allowed to do so.		
9.	Removes and discards gloves. Washes hands.		
10.	Reports and documents incident.		

_____   _____
Date Reviewed   Instructor Signature

_____   _____
Date Performed   Instructor Signature

Responding to vomiting

	Procedure Steps	yes	no
1.	Notifies nurse immediately.		
2.	Puts on gloves.		
3.	Makes sure head is up or turned to one side. Provides a basin and removes it when vomiting has stopped.		

4.	Removes soiled linens or clothes and replaces with fresh ones.		
5.	Measures and notes amount of vomitus if monitoring I&O.		
6.	Flushes vomit down toilet unless vomit is red, has blood in it, or looks like coffee grounds. Washes and stores basin properly.		
7.	Removes and discards gloves. Washes hands.		
8.	Puts on clean gloves.		
9.	Provides comfort to resident.		
10.	Puts soiled linens in proper container.		
11.	Removes and discards gloves. Washes hands again.		
12.	Documents time, amount, color, and consistency of vomitus.		

_____ _____
Date Reviewed   Instructor Signature

_____ _____
Date Performed   Instructor Signature

10
Positioning, Transfers, and Ambulation

Moving a resident up in bed		
Procedure Steps	yes	no
If resident can assist:		
1. Identifies self by name. Identifies resident by name.		
2. Washes hands.		
3. Explains procedure to resident, speaking clearly, slowly, and directly. Maintains face-to-face contact whenever possible.		
4. Provides privacy.		
5. Adjusts the bed to a safe level. Locks bed wheels. Lowers head of bed to make it flat. Moves pillow to head of bed.		

6.	Raises side rail on far side of bed.		
7.	Stands by bed with feet apart, facing resident. Places one arm under resident's shoulders and the other under resident's thighs.		
8.	Asks resident to bend knees, place feet on mattress, and push down with her feet and hands on the count of three.		
9.	On three, shifts body weight and helps resident move toward the head of the bed while she pushes with her feet.		
10.	Positions resident comfortably, arranges pillow and blankets, and returns bed to lowest position.		
11.	Places call light within resident's reach.		
12.	Washes hands.		
13.	Documents procedure.		

_____ _____
Date Reviewed   Instructor Signature

_____ _____
Date Performed   Instructor Signature

When you have help from another person and resident cannot assist:		
1.	Follows steps 1 through 5 above.		
2.	Stands on opposite side of bed from helper. Turns slightly toward head of bed and points foot closest toward head of bed. Stands with feet apart and knees bent.		
3.	Rolls and grasps draw sheet with palms up.		
4.	Shifts weight to back foot and on count of three, both workers shift weight to forward feet while sliding draw sheet toward head of bed.		

		yes	no
5.	Positions resident comfortably, arranges pillow and blankets, unrolls draw sheet, and returns bed to lowest position.		
6.	Places call light within resident's reach.		
7.	Washes hands.		
8.	Documents procedure.		

_____   _____
Date Reviewed   Instructor Signature

_____   _____
Date Performed   Instructor Signature

Moving a resident to the side of the bed

	Procedure Steps	yes	no
1.	Identifies self by name. Identifies resident by name.		
2.	Washes hands.		
3.	Explains procedure to resident, speaking clearly, slowly, and directly. Maintains face-to-face contact whenever possible.		
4.	Provides privacy.		
5.	Adjusts the bed to a safe level. Locks bed wheels. Lowers head of bed.		
6.	Stands on same side of bed where resident will be moved.		
7.	Slides hands under head and shoulders and moves toward self. Slides hands under mid-section and moves toward self. Slides hands under hips and legs and moves toward self.		
8.	Returns bed to lowest position.		
9.	Places call light within resident's reach.		
10.	Washes hands.		
11.	Documents procedure.		

_____   _____
Date Reviewed   Instructor Signature

_____   _____
Date Performed   Instructor Signature

Positioning a resident on the left side

	Procedure Steps	yes	no
1.	Identifies self by name. Identifies resident by name.		
2.	Washes hands.		
3.	Explains procedure to resident, speaking clearly, slowly, and directly. Maintains face-to-face contact whenever possible.		
4.	Provides privacy.		
5.	Adjusts the bed to a safe level. Locks bed wheels. Lowers head of bed.		
6.	Moves resident to right side of bed using proper procedure.		
7.	Raises side rail on left side of bed if bed has rails.		
8.	Crosses resident's right arm over chest and moves left arm out of the way. Crosses right leg over left leg. Stands with feet shoulder-width apart, bends knees, and places one hand on resident's right shoulder and the other on the right hip. Rolls resident toward raised side rail/self.		
9.	Positions resident comfortably using pillows or other supports and checks for alignment.		
10.	Returns bed to lowest position.		
11.	Places call light within resident's reach.		
12.	Washes hands.		
13.	Documents procedure.		

_____   _____
Date Reviewed   Instructor Signature

_____   _____
Date Performed   Instructor Signature

Logrolling a resident

	Procedure Steps	yes	no
1.	Identifies self by name. Identifies resident by name.		
2.	Washes hands.		

Name: _____

		yes	no
3.	Explains procedure to resident, speaking clearly, slowly, and directly. Maintains face-to-face contact whenever possible.		
4.	Provides privacy.		
5.	Adjusts the bed to a safe level. Locks bed wheels. Lowers head of bed.		
6.	Both workers stand on same side of bed, one at the resident's head and shoulders, one near the midsection.		
7.	Places resident's arm across his chest and places pillow between the knees.		
8.	Stands with feet shoulder-width apart, bends knees, and grasps draw sheet on far side.		
9.	Rolls resident toward self on count of three, turning resident as a unit.		
10.	Positions resident comfortably with pillows or supports, and checks for good alignment.		
11.	Returns bed to lowest position.		
12.	Places call light within resident's reach.		
13.	Washes hands.		
14.	Documents procedure.		

_____   _____
Date Reviewed   Instructor Signature

_____   _____
Date Performed   Instructor Signature

Assisting a resident to sit up on side of bed: dangling

	Procedure Steps	yes	no
1.	Identifies self by name. Identifies resident by name.		
2.	Washes hands.		
3.	Explains procedure to resident, speaking clearly, slowly, and directly. Maintains face-to-face contact whenever possible.		

		yes	no
4.	Provides privacy.		
5.	Adjusts the bed to lowest position. Locks bed wheels.		
6.	Raises head of bed to sitting position. Fanfolds top covers to foot of bed and assists resident to turn onto side, facing self.		
7.	Has resident reach across chest with top arm and place hand on edge of bed near opposite shoulder. Asks resident to push down on that hand while swinging legs over the side of bed.		
8.	If resident needs assistance, stands with feet shoulder-width apart and bends knees.		
9.	Places one arm under resident's shoulder blades and the other under his thighs.		
10.	On the count of three, turns resident into sitting position.		
11.	With resident holding onto edge of mattress, puts nonskid shoes on resident.		
12.	Has resident dangle as long as ordered. Does not leave resident alone.		
13.	Removes shoes. Assists resident back into bed by placing one arm around resident's shoulders and the other arm under resident's knees. Slowly swings resident's legs onto the bed. Positions resident comfortably.		
14.	Leaves bed in lowest position.		
15.	Places call light within resident's reach.		
16.	Washes hands.		
17.	Documents procedure.		

_____   _____
Date Reviewed   Instructor Signature

_____   _____
Date Performed   Instructor Signature

Applying a transfer belt

	Procedure Steps	yes	no
1.	Identifies self by name. Identifies resident by name.		
2.	Washes hands.		
3.	Explains procedure to resident, speaking clearly, slowly, and directly. Maintains face-to-face contact whenever possible.		
4.	Provides privacy.		
5.	Adjusts bed to lowest position. Locks bed wheels. Assists resident to sitting position with feet flat on floor.		
6.	Puts on nonskid shoes. Places the belt over the resident's clothing and around the waist. Does not put it over bare skin.		
7.	Tightens the buckle until it is snug. Leaves enough room to insert flat fingers under the belt. Checks to make sure skin is not caught under the belt.		
8.	Positions the buckle off-center in the front or back.		

_____   _____
Date Reviewed   Instructor Signature

_____   _____
Date Performed   Instructor Signature

Transferring a resident from bed to wheelchair

	Procedure Steps	yes	no
1.	Identifies self by name. Identifies resident by name.		
2.	Washes hands.		
3.	Explains procedure to resident, speaking clearly, slowly, and directly. Maintains face-to-face contact whenever possible.		
4.	Provides privacy.		
5.	Places wheelchair on resident's stronger side either at head of the bed, facing foot of the bed or at foot of the bed, facing head of the bed. Removes both footrests close to the bed. Locks wheelchair wheels.		
6.	Raises head of bed and adjusts bed to lowest position. Locks bed wheels.		
7.	Assists resident to sitting position with feet flat on floor. Puts on nonskid shoes.		
8.	Stands in front of resident with feet about shoulder-width apart. Bends knees. Places transfer belt over the resident's clothing and around the waist. Grasps belt on both sides with hands in an upward position.		
9.	Provides instructions to assist with transfer. Braces legs against resident's lower legs. Helps resident stand on count of three.		
10.	Instructs resident to take small steps to the chair while turning back toward chair. Assists resident to pivot to front of chair if necessary.		
11.	Asks resident to put hands on chair armrests and helps resident to lower herself into the chair when chair is touching back of resident's legs.		
12.	Repositions resident with hips touching back of wheelchair. Attaches footrests and places resident's feet on them. Removes transfer belt. Positions resident comfortably, checking for proper alignment and placing robe or blanket over lap.		
13.	Places call light within resident's reach.		

14.	Washes hands.		
15.	Documents procedure.		

Date Reviewed _____ Instructor Signature _____

Date Performed _____ Instructor Signature _____

Transferring a resident from bed to stretcher

	Procedure Steps	yes	no
1.	Identifies self by name. Identifies resident by name.		
2.	Washes hands.		
3.	Explains procedure to resident. Speaks clearly, slowly, and directly. Maintains face-to-face contact whenever possible.		
4.	Provides privacy.		
5.	Lowers head of bed so that it is flat. Locks bed wheels.		
6.	Folds linens to foot of bed and covers resident with blanket.		
7.	Moves resident to side of bed.		
8.	Places stretcher against bed with height of bed equal to or slightly above height of stretcher. Locks stretcher wheels. Moves safety belts out of way.		
9.	Two workers stand on one side of bed opposite stretcher, while two others stand on other side of stretcher. Each worker rolls up sides of draw sheet.		
10.	On count of three, workers lift and move resident to stretcher, centering him or her.		
11.	Places pillow under resident's head. Makes sure resident is still covered. Places safety belts across resident and raises side rails on stretcher.		
12.	Unlocks stretcher's wheels. Moves resident to proper place, staying with resident until another staff member takes over.		

13.	Washes hands.		
14.	Documents procedure.		

Date Reviewed _____ Instructor Signature _____

Date Performed _____ Instructor Signature _____

Transferring a resident using a mechanical lift

	Procedure Steps	yes	no
1.	Identifies self by name. Identifies resident by name.		
2.	Washes hands.		
3.	Explains procedure to resident, speaking clearly, slowly, and directly. Maintains face-to-face contact whenever possible.		
4.	Provides privacy.		
5.	Locks bed wheels. Positions wheelchair next to bed and locks brakes.		
6.	With resident turned to one side of bed, positions sling under resident. Helps resident roll back to middle of bed and spreads out fanfolded edge of sling.		
7.	Positions mechanical lift next to bed, opening the base to its widest point, and pushes base of lift under bed. Positions overhead bar directly over resident.		
8.	Attaches straps to sling properly.		
9.	Raises resident in sling two inches above bed, following manufacturer's instructions. Pauses for resident to gain balance.		
10.	Rolls mechanical lift to position resident over chair or wheelchair. Lifting partner supports and guides resident's body.		
11.	Slowly lowers resident into chair or wheelchair, pushing down gently on resident's knees.		

12.	Undoes straps from overhead bar to sling, removing or leaving sling in place.		
13.	Positions resident comfortably, checking for proper alignment.		
14.	Places call light within resident's reach.		
15.	Washes hands.		
16.	Documents procedure.		

_____   _____
Date Reviewed   Instructor Signature

_____   _____
Date Performed   Instructor Signature

Transferring a resident onto and off of a toilet			
	Procedure Steps	yes	no
1.	Identifies self by name. Identifies resident by name.		
2.	Washes hands.		
3.	Explains procedure to resident. Speaks clearly, slowly, and directly. Maintains face-to-face contact whenever possible.		
4.	Provides privacy.		
5.	Positions wheelchair at right angle to the toilet to face hand bar on resident's stronger side.		
6.	Removes footrests. Locks wheels.		
7.	Puts on gloves.		
8.	Applies a transfer belt over clothing. Grasps the belt with hands in an upward position. Asks resident to push against armrests and to stand. Moves wheelchair out of the way.		
9.	Asks resident to pivot and back up to feel front of toilet with back of her legs.		
10.	Helps resident pull down pants and underwear.		
11.	Helps resident sit down slowly.		

12.	Removes and discards gloves. Washes hands. Leaves bathroom and closes the door.		
13.	When called, returns and washes hands. Dons clean gloves. Assists with perineal care as necessary.		
14.	Cleans and dries resident before pulling up clothing. Removes and discards gloves.		
15.	Helps resident to sink to wash hands. Washes own hands.		
16.	Helps resident into wheelchair and replaces footrests.		
17.	Helps resident leave bathroom.		
18.	Places call light within resident's reach.		
19.	Washes hands again.		
20.	Documents procedure.		

_____   _____
Date Reviewed   Instructor Signature

_____   _____
Date Performed   Instructor Signature

Transferring a resident into a vehicle			
	Procedure Steps	yes	no
1.	Identifies self by name. Identifies resident by name.		
2.	Washes hands.		
3.	Explains procedure to resident. Speaks clearly, slowly, and directly. Maintains face-to-face contact whenever possible.		
4.	Places wheelchair close to vehicle at a 45-degree angle. Opens door on resident's stronger side. Locks wheelchair.		
5.	Asks resident to push against armrests of wheelchair to stand, grasp the vehicle, and pivot foot so that the side of the seat touches back of the legs.		

Name: _____

		yes	no
6.	Helps resident sit in car, lifting one leg, then the other, into the car.		
7.	Positions resident comfortably and secures seat belt.		
8.	Carefully shuts door.		
9.	Returns wheelchair to proper site.		
10.	Washes hands.		
11.	Documents procedure.		

_____   _____
Date Reviewed   Instructor Signature

_____   _____
Date Performed   Instructor Signature

Assisting a resident to ambulate

	Procedure Steps	yes	no
1.	Identifies self by name. Identifies resident by name.		
2.	Washes hands.		
3.	Explains procedure to resident, speaking clearly, slowly, and directly. Maintains face-to-face contact whenever possible.		
4.	Provides privacy.		
5.	Adjusts the bed to lowest position so that feet are flat on the floor. Locks bed wheels. Puts nonskid footwear on resident.		
6.	Stands in front of resident with feet about shoulder-width apart. Bends knees. Places gait belt over the resident's clothing and around the waist. Grasps belt on both sides with hands in an upward position.		
7.	Provides instructions to assist with transfer. Braces legs against resident's lower legs. Helps resident stand on count of three.		
8.	Walks slightly behind and to one side of resident for distance while holding on to gait belt. Asks resident to look forward, not down at floor.		

		yes	no
9.	Observes resident's strength and provides chair if resident becomes tired.		
10.	Removes gait belt and returns resident to bed or a chair. Positions resident comfortably and checks alignment. Leaves bed in lowest position.		
11.	Places call light within resident's reach.		
12.	Washes hands.		
13.	Documents procedure.		

_____   _____
Date Reviewed   Instructor Signature

_____   _____
Date Performed   Instructor Signature

Assisting with ambulation for a resident using a cane, walker, or crutches

	Procedure Steps	yes	no
1.	Identifies self by name. Identifies resident by name.		
2.	Washes hands.		
3.	Explains procedure to resident, speaking clearly, slowly, and directly. Maintains face-to-face contact whenever possible.		
4.	Provides privacy.		
5.	Adjusts the bed to lowest position so that feet are flat on the floor. Locks bed wheels. Puts nonskid footwear on resident.		
6.	Stands in front of resident with feet about shoulder-width apart. Bends knees. Places gait belt over the resident's clothing and around the waist. Grasps belt on both sides with hands in an upward position.		
7.	Provides instructions to assist with transfer. Braces legs against resident's lower legs. Helps resident stand on count of three.		

		yes	no
8.	Helps as needed with ambulation with cane, walker, or crutches, walking slightly behind and to one side while holding on to gait belt.		
9.	Watches for obstacles in the resident's path.		
10.	Lets the resident set the pace, encouraging rest as necessary.		
11.	Removes gait belt and returns resident to bed or a chair. Positions resident comfortably and checks alignment. Leaves bed in lowest position.		
12.	Places call light within resident's reach.		
13.	Washes hands.		
14.	Documents procedure.		

_____   _____
Date Reviewed   Instructor Signature

_____   _____
Date Performed   Instructor Signature

		yes	no
	Completes the paperwork, including an inventory of all personal items.		
	Helps resident put personal items away.		
	Provides fresh water.		
6.	Orients resident to the room and bathroom. Explains how to work equipment.		
7.	Introduces resident to roommate, other residents, and staff.		
8.	Makes resident comfortable and brings family back in.		
9.	Places call light within resident's reach.		
10.	Washes hands.		
11.	Documents procedure.		

_____   _____
Date Reviewed   Instructor Signature

_____   _____
Date Performed   Instructor Signature

11
Admitting, Transferring, and Discharging

Admitting a resident

	Procedure Steps	yes	no
1.	Identifies self by name. Identifies resident by name.		
2.	Washes hands.		
3.	Explains procedure to resident. Speaks clearly, slowly, and directly. Maintains face-to-face contact whenever possible.		
4.	Provides privacy.		
5.	If part of facility procedure, performs the following:		
	Measures resident's height and weight.		
	Measures resident's baseline vital signs.		
	Obtains a urine specimen if required.		

Measuring and recording weight of an ambulatory resident

	Procedure Steps	yes	no
1.	Identifies self by name. Identifies resident by name.		
2.	Washes hands.		
3.	Explains procedure to resident. Speaks clearly, slowly, and directly. Maintains face-to-face contact whenever possible.		
4.	Provides privacy.		
5.	Makes sure resident is wearing fastened nonskid shoes. Starts with scale balanced at zero before weighing resident.		
6.	Helps resident to step onto the center of the scale. Makes sure resident is not holding, touching, or leaning against anything.		
7.	Determines resident's weight.		
8.	Helps resident off of scale before recording weight.		

9.	Washes hands.		
10.	Records weight.		
11.	Places call light within resident's reach.		
12.	Documents procedure.		

_____   _____
Date Reviewed   Instructor Signature

_____   _____
Date Performed   Instructor Signature

Measuring and recording height of an ambulatory resident

	Procedure Steps	yes	no
1.	Identifies self by name. Identifies resident by name.		
2.	Washes hands.		
3.	Explains procedure to resident. Speaks clearly, slowly, and directly. Maintains face-to-face contact whenever possible.		
4.	Provides privacy.		
5.	Makes sure resident is wearing fastened nonskid shoes. Helps resident step onto the scale, facing away from scale.		
6.	Asks resident to stand straight. Helps as needed.		
7.	Pulls up measuring rod from back of scale. Gently lowers measuring rod until it rests flat on resident's head.		
8.	Determines resident's height.		
9.	Helps resident off scale before recording height.		
10.	Washes hands.		
11.	Records height.		
12.	Places call light within resident's reach.		
13.	Documents procedure.		

_____   _____
Date Reviewed   Instructor Signature

_____   _____
Date Performed   Instructor Signature

Transferring a resident

	Procedure Steps	yes	no
1.	Identifies self by name. Identifies resident by name.		
2.	Washes hands.		
3.	Explains procedure to resident. Speaks clearly, slowly, and directly. Maintains face-to-face contact whenever possible.		
4.	Collects the items to be transferred and takes them to the new location.		
5.	Helps resident into the wheelchair or stretcher. Takes him to proper area.		
6.	Introduces new residents and staff.		
7.	Helps resident to put personal items away.		
8.	Makes resident comfortable. Places call light within resident's reach.		
9.	Washes hands.		
10.	Documents procedure.		

_____   _____
Date Reviewed   Instructor Signature

_____   _____
Date Performed   Instructor Signature

Discharging a resident

	Procedure Steps	yes	no
1.	Identifies self by name. Identifies resident by name.		
2.	Washes hands.		
3.	Explains procedure to resident. Speaks clearly, slowly, and directly. Maintains face-to-face contact whenever possible.		
4.	Provides privacy.		
5.	Measures vital signs.		
6.	Compares the checklist to the items there. If all items are there, asks resident to sign.		

		yes	no
7.	Puts items to be taken onto cart and takes them to pickup area.		
8.	Helps resident dress and then into the wheelchair or stretcher.		
9.	Helps resident say goodbye to the staff and residents.		
10.	Takes resident to the pickup area and assists into vehicle.		
11.	Washes hands.		
12.	Documents procedure.		

_____   _____
Date Reviewed   Instructor Signature

_____   _____
Date Performed   Instructor Signature

12
The Resident's Unit

Making an occupied bed			
	Procedure Steps	yes	no
1.	Identifies self by name. Identifies resident by name.		
2.	Washes hands.		
3.	Explains procedure to resident, speaking clearly, slowly, and directly. Maintains face-to-face contact whenever possible.		
4.	Provides privacy.		
5.	Places clean linen on clean surface within reach (e.g., bedside stand, overbed table, or chair).		
6.	Adjusts the bed to a safe level, usually waist high. Lowers head of bed. Locks bed wheels.		
7.	Puts on gloves.		
8.	Loosens top linen from working side. Unfolds bath blanket over top sheet to cover resident and removes top sheet.		
9.	Raises side rail on far side of bed and turns resident onto her side, toward self and raised side rail.		
10.	Loosens bottom soiled linen, mattress pad, and absorbent pad on working side.		
11.	Rolls bottom soiled linen toward resident, soiled side inside. Tucks it snugly against the resident's back.		
12.	Places mattress pad on the bed. Places and tucks in clean bottom linen, finishing with no wrinkles. Makes hospital corners if necessary.		
13.	Smooths bottom sheet out toward the resident. Rolls extra material toward resident and tucks it under resident's body.		
14.	Places absorbent pad, if using, and centers it. Tucks side near self under mattress and smooths it out toward resident.		
15.	Places draw sheet if using. Smooths and tucks as with other bedding.		
16.	Raises side rail on working side and helps resident to turn onto clean bottom sheet, toward self.		
17.	Goes to far side and lowers side rail. Loosens soiled linen. Rolls linen from head to the foot of bed, avoiding contact with skin or clothes. Places it in hamper or bag.		
18.	Pulls through and tucks in clean bottom linen just like other side, finishing with bottom sheet free of wrinkles.		
19.	Asks resident to turn onto her back, keeping resident covered. Raises side rail nearest self.		
20.	Unfolds top sheet and places it over resident. Asks resident to hold onto top sheet and slips blanket or old sheet out from underneath. Puts it in hamper or bag.		

Name: _____

21.	Places a blanket over the top sheet, matching the top edges. Tucks bottom edges of top sheet and blanket under mattress, making hospital corners on each side. Loosens top linens over resident's feet. Folds top sheet over the blanket about six inches.		
22.	Removes pillows and pillowcase. Places pillowcases in hamper or bag.		
23.	Removes and discards gloves. Washes hands.		
24.	Places clean pillowcases on pillows. Places them under resident's head with open end away from door.		
25.	Returns bed to lowest position. Leaves side rails in ordered position.		
26.	Places call light within resident's reach.		
27.	Takes hamper or bag to proper area.		
28.	Washes hands.		
29.	Documents procedure.		

_____   _____
Date Reviewed   Instructor Signature

_____   _____
Date Performed   Instructor Signature

5.	Loosens soiled linen and rolls it from head to foot of bed. Avoids contact with skin or clothes. Places it in a hamper or bag. Removes pillow and pillowcase and places in the hamper.		
6.	Removes and discards gloves. Washes hands.		
7.	Remakes bed, spreading mattress pad and bottom sheet, tucking under. Makes hospital corners. Puts on absorbent pad and draw sheet, smooths, and tucks under sides of bed.		
8.	Places top sheet, blanket, and bedspread, centering them. Tucks under end of bed and makes hospital corners. Folds down top sheet over the blanket about six inches.		
9.	Puts on clean pillowcases. Replaces pillows.		
10.	Returns bed to its lowest position.		
11.	Takes hamper or bag to proper area.		
12.	Washes hands.		
13.	Documents procedure.		

_____   _____
Date Reviewed   Instructor Signature

_____   _____
Date Performed   Instructor Signature

Making an unoccupied bed

	Procedure Steps	yes	no
1.	Washes hands.		
2.	Places clean linen on clean surface within reach (e.g., bedside stand, overbed table, or chair).		
3.	Adjusts the bed to a safe level. Puts bed in flattest position. Locks bed wheels.		
4.	Puts on gloves.		

Making a surgical bed

	Procedure Steps	yes	no
1.	Washes hands.		
2.	Places clean linen on clean surface within reach (e.g., bedside stand, overbed table, or chair).		
3.	Adjusts the bed to a safe level. Locks bed wheels.		
4.	Puts on gloves.		

5.	Loosens soiled linen and rolls it from head to foot of bed. Avoids contact with skin or clothes. Places it in hamper or bag.		
6.	Removes and discards gloves. Washes hands.		
7.	Makes an unoccupied, closed bed, with bedding left up.		
8.	Loosens linens on side of bed that is away from door (where stretcher will be).		
9.	Fanfolds linens lengthwise to the side away from door.		
10.	Puts on clean pillowcases. Replaces pillows.		
11.	Leaves bed in locked position with both side rails down.		
12.	Makes sure pathway to bed is clear.		
13.	Takes hamper or bag to proper area.		
14.	Washes hands.		
15.	Documents procedure.		

_____   _____
Date Reviewed   Instructor Signature

_____   _____
Date Performed   Instructor Signature

13
Personal Care Skills

Giving a complete bed bath			
	Procedure Steps	yes	no
1.	Identifies self by name. Identifies resident by name.		
2.	Washes hands.		
3.	Explains procedure to resident, speaking clearly, slowly, and directly. Maintains face-to-face contact whenever possible.		
4.	Provides privacy.		
5.	Adjusts the bed to a safe level. Locks bed wheels.		

6.	Places blanket over resident and removes top bedding and gown while keeping resident covered.		
7.	Fills basin and checks temperature (no higher than 105°F). Has resident test water temperature and adjusts if necessary.		
8.	Puts on gloves.		
9.	Asks and helps resident to participate in washing.		
10.	Uncovers only one part of the body at a time. Places a towel under the body part being washed.		
11.	Washes, rinses, and dries one part of the body at a time. Starts at the head, works down, and completes front first. Uses a clean area of washcloth for each stroke.		
	Eyes, Face, Ears, and Neck: Washes face with wet washcloth (no soap) beginning with the eyes, using a different area of the washcloth for each eye, washing inner area to outer area. Uses a different area of the washcloth for each stroke. Washes the face from the middle outward, using firm but gentle strokes. Washes ears, behind the ears, and the neck. Rinses and pats dry.		
	Arms and Axillae: Washes upper arm and underarm. Uses long strokes from the shoulder down to the wrist. Rinses and pats dry. Repeats for other arm.		
	Hands: Washes one hand in a basin. Cleans under nails. Rinses and pats dry. Gives nail care. Repeats for other hand. Applies lotion if ordered.		

Name: _____

	Chest: Places towel across the chest and pulls blanket down to waist. Lifts the towel only enough to wash the chest, rinse it, and pat dry. For a female resident: washes, rinses, and dries breasts and under breasts.		
	Abdomen: Folds blanket down so that pubic area is still covered. Washes abdomen, rinses, and pats dry. Covers with towel, pulls blanket up to the chin, and removes towel.		
	Legs and Feet: Exposes one leg and places towel under it. Washes the thigh. Uses long, downward strokes. Rinses and pats dry. Does the same from the knee to the ankle. Washes the foot and between the toes in a basin. Rinses foot and pats dry, making sure area between toes is dry. Gives nail care if it has been assigned. Applies lotion if ordered but not between the toes. Repeats steps for other leg and foot.		
	Back: Helps resident move to the center of the bed. Raises side rail on far side and asks resident to turn onto side, toward raised side rail. Goes to working side. Folds blanket away from back and washes back with long, downward strokes. Rinses and pats dry. Applies lotion if ordered.		
12.	Places towel under buttocks and thighs and helps resident turn onto his back. Removes and discards gloves. Washes hands and dons clean gloves.		

13.	**Perineal area and buttocks**: Changes bath water. Washes, rinses, and dries perineal area, working from front to back, using a clean area of the washcloth for each stroke. After cleaning perineal area, helps turn resident on his or her side, and washes, rinses, and dries buttocks and anal area without contaminating the perineal area.		
14.	Covers resident. Empties, rinses, and dries bath basin. Places basin in dirty supply area or returns to storage. Places soiled clothing and linens in proper containers.		
15.	Removes and discards gloves. Washes hands.		
16.	Puts clean clothes on resident and assists with grooming as necessary.		
17.	Returns bed to lowest position.		
18.	Places call light within resident's reach.		
19.	Washes hands.		
20.	Documents procedure.		

_____   _____
Date Reviewed   Instructor Signature

_____   _____
Date Performed   Instructor Signature

Giving a back rub

	Procedure Steps	yes	no
1.	Identifies self by name. Identifies resident by name.		
2.	Washes hands.		
3.	Explains procedure to resident, speaking clearly, slowly, and directly. Maintains face-to-face contact whenever possible.		
4.	Provides privacy.		
5.	Adjusts the bed to a safe level. Lowers head of bed. Locks bed wheels.		

6.	Positions resident in lateral or prone position. Covers resident with blanket and folds back bed covers, exposing resident's back to the top of the buttocks.		
7.	Warms lotion and hands. Pours lotion onto hands and rubs hands together.		
8.	Starting at the upper part of the buttocks, makes long, smooth, upward strokes with both hands. Circles hands up along spine, shoulders, and then back down along the outer edges of the back. At buttocks, makes another circle back up to the shoulders. Repeats for three to five minutes.		
9.	Starting at the base of the spine, makes kneading motions using the first two fingers and thumb of each hand. Circles hands up along spine, circling at shoulders and buttocks.		
10.	Gently massages bony areas. Massages around any white, red, purple areas, rather than on them.		
11.	Lets resident know when back rub is almost completed. Finishes with long, smooth strokes.		
12.	Dries the back.		
13.	Removes blanket and towel, assists resident with getting dressed, and positions resident comfortably.		
14.	Stores supplies and places soiled clothing and linens in proper containers.		
15.	Returns bed to lowest position.		
16.	Places call light within resident's reach.		
17.	Washes hands.		

18.	Documents procedure.		

_____ _____
Date Reviewed   Instructor Signature

_____ _____
Date Performed   Instructor Signature

Shampooing hair

	Procedure Steps	yes	no
1.	Identifies self by name. Identifies resident by name.		
2.	Washes hands.		
3.	Explains procedure to resident, speaking clearly, slowly, and directly. Maintains face-to-face contact whenever possible.		
4.	Provides privacy.		
5.	Tests water temperature (no higher than 105°F). Has resident test water temperature and adjusts if necessary.		
6.	Positions resident at sink or in bed and wets hair.		
7.	Applies shampoo and massages scalp.		
8.	Rinses hair thoroughly. Repeats. Uses conditioner if requested.		
9.	Wraps resident's hair.		
10.	Removes towel and combs or brushes hair.		
11.	Dries and styles hair.		
12.	Returns bed to lowest position if adjusted.		
13.	Places call light within resident's reach.		
14.	Washes and stores equipment.		
15.	Washes hands.		
16.	Documents procedure.		

_____ _____
Date Reviewed   Instructor Signature

_____ _____
Date Performed   Instructor Signature

Giving a shower or tub bath

	Procedure Steps	yes	no
1.	Washes hands. Places equipment in area. Puts on gloves. Cleans area. Places bucket under shower chair.		
2.	Removes and discards gloves. Washes hands.		
3.	Goes to resident's room. Identifies self by name. Identifies resident by name. Washes hands.		
4.	Explains procedure to resident, speaking clearly, slowly, and directly. Maintains face-to-face contact whenever possible.		
5.	Provides privacy.		
6.	Helps resident put on nonskid footwear and transports to shower or tub room.		
7.	Washes hands and puts on clean gloves. Helps resident remove clothing and shoes.		
	For a shower:		
8.	Places shower chair in position. Locks wheels. Transfers resident into chair.		
9.	Turns on water. Tests water temperature (no higher than 105°F). Has resident test water temperature and adjusts if necessary.		
10.	Unlocks chair and moves it into stall. Locks chair wheels.		
11.	Stays with resident during procedure. Lets resident wash as much as possible. Helps to wash his face. Helps to shampoo and rinse hair.		
12.	Helps to wash and rinse entire body, moving from head to toe.		
13.	Turns off water. Unlocks wheels and rolls resident out of shower.		
	For a tub bath:		
8.	Transfers resident onto tub lift or helps resident into bath.		
9.	Fills tub halfway with warm water. Tests water temperature (no higher than 105°F). Has resident test water temperature and adjusts if necessary.		
10.	Stays with resident during procedure. Lets resident wash as much as possible. Helps to wash his face. Helps to shampoo and rinse hair.		
11.	Helps to wash and rinse entire body, moving from head to toe.		
12.	Drains tub and covers resident with the bath blanket.		
13.	Helps resident out of tub and onto a chair.		
	Final steps:		
14.	Gives resident a towel and helps to pat dry all areas of body. Applies lotion and deodorant as needed.		
15.	Places soiled clothing and linen in proper containers.		
16.	Removes and discards gloves.		
17.	Washes hands.		
18.	Helps resident dress, comb hair, and put on footwear. Returns resident to his or her room.		
19.	Places call light within resident's reach.		
20.	Documents procedure.		

_____   _____
Date Reviewed   Instructor Signature

_____   _____
Date Performed   Instructor Signature

Providing fingernail care

	Procedure Steps	yes	no
1.	Identifies self by name. Identifies resident by name.		
2.	Washes hands.		
3.	Explains procedure to resident, speaking clearly, slowly, and directly. Maintains face-to-face contact whenever possible.		

4.	Provides privacy.		
5.	Adjusts the bed to a safe level. Locks bed wheels.		
6.	Fills basin halfway with warm water. Tests water temperature (no higher than 105°F). Has resident test water temperature and adjusts if necessary.		
7.	Puts on gloves.		
8.	Soaks all 10 fingertips for at least five minutes.		
9.	Removes hands from water. Washes hands with soapy washcloth. Rinses. Pats dry resident's hands with a towel, including between fingers.		
10.	Places resident's hands on towel and gently cleans under each fingernail with orangewood stick. Wipes stick on towel after cleaning and washes resident's hands again. Dries hands thoroughly, especially between fingers.		
11.	Shapes fingernails in a curve with an emery board or nail file. Finishes with nails free of rough edges. Applies lotion.		
12.	Empties, rinses, and dries basin. Places basin in designated area or returns to storage. Places soiled clothing and linens in proper containers.		
13.	Removes and discards gloves and washes hands.		
14.	Returns bed to lowest position.		
15.	Places call light within resident's reach.		
16.	Washes hands.		
17.	Documents procedure.		

_____   _____
Date Reviewed   Instructor Signature

_____   _____
Date Performed   Instructor Signature

Providing foot care

	Procedure Steps	yes	no
1.	Identifies self by name. Identifies resident by name.		
2.	Washes hands.		
3.	Explains procedure to resident, speaking clearly, slowly, and directly. Maintains face-to-face contact whenever possible.		
4.	Provides privacy.		
5.	Adjusts the bed to a safe level. Locks bed wheels.		
6.	Fills basin halfway with warm water. Tests water temperature (no higher than 105°F). Has resident test water temperature and adjusts if necessary.		
7.	Places basin at comfortable position. Puts on gloves.		
8.	Removes socks. Completely submerges feet in water and soaks feet for 10 to 20 minutes, adding warm water as necessary.		
9.	Puts soap on washcloth. Removes one foot from water. Washes entire foot, including between the toes and around nail beds.		
10.	Rinses and dries entire foot, including between the toes.		
11.	Repeats steps for other foot.		
12.	Applies lotion except for between the toes. Helps put on clean socks.		
13.	Empties, rinses, and dries basin. Places basin in designated area or returns to storage. Places soiled clothing and linens in proper containers.		
14.	Removes and discards gloves and washes hands.		
15.	Returns bed to lowest position.		
16.	Places call light within resident's reach.		

		yes	no
17.	Washes hands.		
18.	Documents procedure.		

_____ _____
Date Reviewed   Instructor Signature

_____ _____
Date Performed   Instructor Signature

Shaving a resident

	Procedure Steps	yes	no
1.	Identifies self by name. Identifies resident by name.		
2.	Washes hands.		
3.	Explains procedure to resident, speaking clearly, slowly, and directly. Maintains face-to-face contact whenever possible.		
4.	Provides privacy.		
5.	Adjusts bed to a safe level. Locks bed wheels. Raises head of bed so that resident is sitting up.		
6.	Places towel across resident's chest, under the chin.		
7.	Puts on gloves.		
	If using a safety or disposable razor:		
8.	Softens beard and lathers face. Shaves in direction of hair growth, using downward strokes on face and upward strokes on neck. Rinses blade often. Rinses and dries face. Offers mirror.		
	If using an electric razor:		
8.	Cleans razor. Turns on, pulls skin taut, and shaves with smooth, even movements. With foil shaver, shaves beard with back and forth motion in direction of beard growth. Shaves beard in circular motion with three-head shaver. Shaves chin and under chin. Offers mirror.		

	Final steps:	yes	no
9.	Applies aftershave if resident desires.		
10.	Puts towel and linens in proper container. Cleans and stores equipment.		
11.	Removes and discards gloves. Washes hands.		
12.	Returns bed to lowest position.		
13.	Places call light within resident's reach.		
14.	Documents procedure.		

_____ _____
Date Reviewed   Instructor Signature

_____ _____
Date Performed   Instructor Signature

Combing or brushing hair

	Procedure Steps	yes	no
1.	Identifies self by name. Identifies resident by name.		
2.	Washes hands.		
3.	Explains procedure to resident, speaking clearly, slowly, and directly. Maintains face-to-face contact whenever possible.		
4.	Provides privacy.		
5.	Adjusts the bed to a safe level. Locks bed wheels. Raises head of bed so that resident is sitting up.		
6.	Places towel under head or around shoulders. Removes hair pins, hair ties, and clips.		
7.	If hair is tangled, detangles gently.		
8.	Brushes hair in two-inch sections at a time.		
9.	Styles hair in the way the resident prefers. Offers a mirror to resident.		
10.	Cleans and stores equipment. Puts soiled linen in proper containers. Returns bed to lowest position.		

Name: _____

		yes	no
11.	Places call light within resident's reach.		
12.	Washes hands.		
13.	Documents procedure.		

```
_____        _____
Date Reviewed              Instructor Signature

_____        _____
Date Performed             Instructor Signature
```

Dressing a resident

	Procedure Steps	yes	no
	When putting on all items, moves resident's body gently and naturally. Avoids force and overextension of limbs and joints.		
1.	Identifies self by name. Identifies resident by name.		
2.	Washes hands.		
3.	Explains procedure to resident, speaking clearly, slowly, and directly. Maintains face-to-face contact whenever possible.		
4.	Provides privacy.		
5.	Adjusts bed to a safe level. Locks bed wheels. Raises head of bed so that resident is sitting up.		
6.	Asks resident which outfit she would like to wear. Dresses her in outfit of choice.		
7.	Puts on gloves if resident has non-intact skin. Places blanket over resident and folds back top bedding to foot of bed.		
8.	Removes resident's gown or top clothing while keeping resident covered. Takes clothes off stronger side first when undressing. Then removes clothes from weaker side. Places clothing in hamper. Moves blanket down to cover lower body.		

		yes	no
9.	Places bra on resident if worn. Places top on resident. Helps resident put the weaker arm through the sleeve before placing garment on stronger arm.		
10.	Removes blanket and places in container. Helps resident put on skirt or pants, putting weaker leg in first.		
11.	Rolls on sock on weaker foot, then stronger foot. Puts on non-skid footwear.		
12.	Finishes with resident dressed appropriately. Makes sure clothing is right-side-out and zippers and buttons are fastened.		
13.	Returns bed to lowest position.		
14.	Places call light within resident's reach.		
15.	Washes hands.		
16.	Documents procedure.		

```
_____        _____
Date Reviewed              Instructor Signature

_____        _____
Date Performed             Instructor Signature
```

Providing oral care

	Procedure Steps	yes	no
1.	Identifies self by name. Identifies resident by name.		
2.	Washes hands.		
3.	Explains procedure to resident, speaking clearly, slowly, and directly. Maintains face-to-face contact whenever possible.		
4.	Provides privacy.		
5.	Adjusts bed to a safe level. Raises head of bed so that resident is sitting upright. Locks bed wheels.		
6.	Puts on gloves.		
7.	Places clothing protector or towel across resident's chest.		

		yes	no
8.	Wets brush and puts on small amount of toothpaste.		
9.	Cleans entire mouth (including tongue and all surfaces of teeth and gumline), using gentle strokes. First brushes inner, outer, and chewing surfaces of upper teeth, then lower teeth. Brushes tongue.		
10.	Holds emesis basin to resident's chin. Has resident rinse mouth with water and spit into emesis basin. Wipes resident's mouth and removes towel.		
11.	Rinses toothbrush and places in proper container. Empties, rinses, and dries basin. Places basin in designated area or returns to storage. Places soiled clothing and linens in proper containers.		
12.	Removes and discards gloves. Washes hands.		
13.	Returns bed to lowest position.		
14.	Places call light within resident's reach.		
15.	Washes hands.		
16.	Documents procedure.		

_____   _____
Date Reviewed   Instructor Signature

_____   _____
Date Performed   Instructor Signature

Providing oral care for the unconscious resident

	Procedure Steps	yes	no
1.	Identifies self by name. Identifies resident by name.		
2.	Washes hands.		
3.	Explains procedure to resident, speaking clearly, slowly, and directly. Maintains face-to-face contact whenever possible.		
4.	Provides privacy.		
5.	Adjusts bed to a safe level. Locks bed wheels.		
6.	Puts on gloves.		
7.	Turns resident on side or turns head to the side and places a towel under his cheek and chin. Places an emesis basin next to the cheek and chin.		
8.	Holds mouth open with tongue depressor.		
9.	Dips swab in cleaning solution. Squeezes out excess solution. Wipes teeth, gums, tongue, and inside surfaces of mouth, changing swab frequently. Repeats until the mouth is clean.		
10.	Rinses with clean swab dipped in water. Squeezes out excess water first.		
11.	Removes the towel and basin. Pats lips or face dry if needed. Applies lip moisturizer.		
12.	Empties, rinses, and dries basin. Places basin in designated area or returns to storage. Places soiled clothing and linens in proper containers.		
13.	Removes and discards gloves. Washes hands.		
14.	Returns bed to lowest position.		
15.	Places call light within resident's reach.		
16.	Washes hands.		
17.	Documents procedure.		

_____   _____
Date Reviewed   Instructor Signature

_____   _____
Date Performed   Instructor Signature

Flossing teeth

	Procedure Steps	yes	no
1.	Identifies self by name. Identifies resident by name.		
2.	Washes hands.		

3.	Explains procedure to resident, speaking clearly, slowly, and directly. Maintains face-to-face contact whenever possible.		
4.	Provides privacy.		
5.	Adjusts bed to a safe level. Raises head of bed so that resident is sitting up. Locks bed wheels.		
6.	Puts on gloves.		
7.	Wraps floss around index fingers.		
8.	Flosses teeth, starting with back and moving to gum line.		
9.	Uses clean area of floss after every two teeth.		
10.	Offers water periodically and offers a towel when done.		
11.	Discards floss. Empties, rinses, and dries basin. Places basin in designated area or returns to storage. Places soiled clothing and linens in proper containers.		
12.	Removes and discards gloves. Washes hands.		
13.	Returns bed to lowest position.		
14.	Places call light within resident's reach.		
15.	Washes hands.		
16.	Documents procedure.		

Date Reviewed _____   Instructor Signature _____

Date Performed _____   Instructor Signature _____

Cleaning and storing dentures		
Procedure Steps	yes	no
1. Washes hands.		
2. Puts on gloves.		
3. Lines sink/basin with towels and partially fills with water.		
4. Rinses dentures in clean cool running water before brushing them.		

5.	Applies toothpaste or cleanser to toothbrush.		
6.	Brushes dentures on all surfaces.		
7.	Rinses all surfaces of dentures under clean cool running water.		
8.	Rinses denture cup before placing clean dentures in it.		
9.	Places dentures in clean, labeled denture cup with solution or cool water, or returns dentures to resident.		
10.	Rinses denture brush and places in proper container. Cleans, dries, and returns the equipment to proper storage. Drains sink and places soiled linens in proper containers.		
11.	Removes and discards gloves. Washes hands.		
12.	Documents procedure.		

Date Reviewed _____   Instructor Signature _____

Date Performed _____   Instructor Signature _____

14
Basic Nursing Skills

Measuring and recording an oral temperature		
Procedure Steps	yes	no
1. Identifies self by name. Identifies resident by name.		
2. Washes hands.		
3. Explains procedure to resident, speaking clearly, slowly, and directly. Maintains face-to-face contact whenever possible.		
4. Provides privacy.		
5. Puts on gloves.		
6. **Digital thermometer:** Puts on disposable sheath. Turns on thermometer and waits until ready sign appears.		

Name: _____

	Electronic thermometer: Removes probe from base unit and puts on probe cover.		
	Mercury-free thermometer: Holds thermometer by stem. Shakes thermometer down to below the lowest number.		
7.	**Digital thermometer:** Inserts end of digital thermometer into resident's mouth, under tongue and to one side.		
	Electronic thermometer: Inserts end of electronic thermometer into resident's mouth, under tongue and to one side.		
	Mercury-free thermometer: Puts on disposable sheath if available. Inserts bulb end of thermometer into resident's mouth, under tongue and to one side.		
8.	**For all thermometers:** Instructs resident on how to hold thermometer in mouth.		
	Digital thermometer: Leaves in place until thermometer blinks or beeps.		
	Electronic thermometer: Leaves in place until tone or light signals temperature has been read.		
	Mercury-free thermometer: Leaves thermometer in place for at least three minutes.		
9.	**Digital thermometer:** Removes thermometer. Reads temperature on display screen and remembers reading.		
	Electronic thermometer: Reads temperature on display screen and remembers reading.		
	Mercury-free thermometer: Removes thermometer. Wipes with tissue from stem to bulb or removes sheath. Discards tissue or sheath. Reads temperature and remembers reading.		

10.	**Digital thermometer:** Removes and discards sheath with a tissue. Replaces thermometer in case.		
	Electronic thermometer: Presses the eject button to discard the cover. Returns probe to holder.		
	Mercury-free thermometer: Cleans thermometer according to policy. Rinses and dries thermometer. Returns to case.		
11.	Removes and discards gloves.		
12	Washes hands.		
13.	Documents temperature, date, time, and method used.		
14.	Places call light within resident's reach.		

_____ _____
Date Reviewed   Instructor Signature

_____ _____
Date Performed   Instructor Signature

Measuring and recording a rectal temperature

	Procedure Steps	yes	no
1.	Identifies self by name. Identifies resident by name.		
2.	Washes hands.		
3.	Explains procedure to resident, speaking clearly, slowly, and directly. Maintains face-to-face contact whenever possible.		
4.	Provides privacy.		
5.	Adjusts bed to safe level. Locks bed wheels.		
6.	Helps resident to left-lying position.		
7.	Folds back linens to expose only rectal area.		
8.	Puts on gloves.		
9.	**Digital thermometer:** Puts on disposable sheath. Turns on thermometer and waits until ready sign appears.		

#	Procedure Steps		
	Electronic thermometer: Removes probe from base unit and puts on probe cover.		
	Mercury-free thermometer: Holds thermometer by stem. Shakes thermometer down to below the lowest number.		
10.	Applies a small amount of lubricant to tip of bulb or probe cover.		
11.	Separates buttocks. Gently inserts thermometer into rectum 1/2 to 1 inch. Replaces sheet over buttocks. Holds onto thermometer at all times while taking temperature.		
12.	**Digital thermometer:** Leaves thermometer in place until thermometer blinks or beeps.		
	Electronic thermometer: Leaves in place until tone or light signals temperature has been read.		
	Mercury-free thermometer: Leaves thermometer in place for at least three minutes.		
13.	Removes thermometer and wipes thermometer with tissue from stem to bulb or removes sheath. Discards tissue or sheath.		
14.	Reads temperature and remembers reading.		
15.	**Digital thermometer:** Cleans thermometer according to policy. Replaces thermometer in case.		
	Electronic thermometer: Presses the eject button to discard the cover. Returns probe to holder.		
	Mercury-free thermometer: Cleans thermometer according to policy. Rinses and dries thermometer. Returns to case.		
16.	Removes and discards gloves.		
17.	Washes hands.		
18.	Documents temperature, date, time, and method used.		
19.	Places call light within resident's reach.		

Date Reviewed _____ Instructor Signature _____

Date Performed _____ Instructor Signature _____

Measuring and recording a tympanic temperature

#	Procedure Steps	yes	no
1.	Identifies self by name. Identifies resident by name.		
2.	Washes hands.		
3.	Explains procedure to resident, speaking clearly, slowly, and directly. Maintains face-to-face contact whenever possible.		
4.	Provides privacy.		
5.	Puts on gloves.		
6.	Places disposable sheath over earpiece of thermometer.		
7.	Positions resident's head properly and pulls up and back on the outside edge of the ear. Inserts covered probe and presses the button.		
8.	Holds thermometer in place until it beeps.		
9.	Reads temperature and remembers reading.		
10.	Discards sheath and stores thermometer properly.		
11.	Removes and discards gloves.		
12.	Washes hands.		
13.	Documents temperature, date, time, and method used.		
14.	Places call light within resident's reach.		

Date Reviewed _____ Instructor Signature _____

Date Performed _____ Instructor Signature _____

Measuring and recording an axillary temperature

	Procedure Steps	yes	no
1.	Identifies self by name. Identifies resident by name.		
2.	Washes hands.		
3.	Explains procedure to resident, speaking clearly, slowly, and directly. Maintains face-to-face contact whenever possible.		
4.	Provides privacy.		
5.	Puts on gloves.		
6.	Removes resident's arm from sleeve and wipes axillary area with tissues.		
7.	**Digital thermometer:** Puts on disposable sheath. Turns on thermometer and waits until ready sign appears.		
	Electronic thermometer: Removes probe from base unit and puts on probe cover.		
	Mercury-free thermometer: Holds thermometer by stem. Shakes thermometer down to below the lowest number.		
8.	Positions thermometer in center of armpit and folds resident's arm over chest.		
9.	**Digital thermometer:** Leaves in place until thermometer blinks or beeps.		
	Electronic thermometer: Leaves in place until tone or light signals temperature has been read.		
	Mercury-free thermometer: Holds thermometer in place for eight to ten minutes.		
10.	**Digital thermometer:** Removes thermometer. Reads temperature on display screen and remembers reading.		
	Electronic thermometer: Reads temperature on display screen and remembers reading.		

		yes	no
	Mercury-free thermometer: Removes thermometer. Wipes with tissue from stem to bulb or removes sheath. Discards tissue or sheath. Reads temperature and remembers reading.		
11.	**Digital thermometer:** Removes and discards sheath with a tissue. Replaces thermometer in case.		
	Electronic thermometer: Presses the eject button to discard the cover. Returns probe to holder.		
	Mercury-free thermometer: Cleans thermometer according to policy. Rinses and dries thermometer. Returns to case.		
12.	Removes and discards gloves.		
13.	Washes hands.		
14.	Puts resident's arm back into sleeve.		
15.	Documents temperature, date, time, and method used.		
16.	Places call light within resident's reach.		

_____ _____
Date Reviewed   Instructor Signature

_____ _____
Date Performed   Instructor Signature

Counting and recording apical pulse

	Procedure Steps	yes	no
1.	Identifies self by name. Identifies resident by name.		
2.	Washes hands.		
3.	Explains procedure to resident, speaking clearly, slowly, and directly. Maintains face-to-face contact whenever possible.		
4.	Provides privacy.		

5.	Before using stethoscope, wipes diaphragm and earpieces with alcohol wipes. Fits earpieces of stethoscope snugly in ears and places metal diaphragm on left side of chest, just below the nipple.		
6.	Counts heartbeats for one full minute.		
7.	Washes hands.		
8.	Documents pulse rate, date, time, and method used. Notes any irregularities in rhythm.		
9.	Cleans earpieces and diaphragm of stethoscope. Stores stethoscope.		
10.	Places call light within resident's reach.		

_____   _____
Date Reviewed   Instructor Signature

_____   _____
Date Performed   Instructor Signature

Counting and recording radial pulse and counting and recording respirations

	Procedure Steps	yes	no
1.	Identifies self by name. Identifies resident by name.		
2.	Washes hands.		
3.	Explains procedure to resident, speaking clearly, slowly, and directly. Maintains face-to-face contact whenever possible.		
4.	Provides privacy.		
5.	Places fingertips of index finger and middle finger on the thumb side of resident's wrist to locate radial pulse.		
6.	Counts beats for one full minute.		
7.	Keeping fingertips on resident's wrist, counts respirations for one full minute.		
8.	Washes hands.		

9.	Documents pulse rate, date, time, and method used. Documents respiratory rate and the pattern or character of breathing.		
10.	Places call light within resident's reach.		

_____   _____
Date Reviewed   Instructor Signature

_____   _____
Date Performed   Instructor Signature

Measuring and recording blood pressure (one-step method)

	Procedure Steps	yes	no
1.	Identifies self by name. Identifies resident by name.		
2.	Washes hands.		
3.	Explains procedure to resident, speaking clearly, slowly, and directly. Maintains face-to-face contact whenever possible.		
4.	Provides privacy.		
5.	Wipes diaphragm and earpieces of stethoscope with alcohol wipes.		
6.	Asks resident to roll up sleeve. Positions resident's arm with palm up. The arm should be level with the heart.		
7.	With the valve open, squeezes the cuff to make sure it is completely deflated.		
8.	Places blood pressure cuff snugly on resident's upper arm, with the center of the cuff with sensor/arrow placed over the brachial artery.		
9.	Locates the brachial pulse with fingertips. Places earpieces of stethoscope in ears and diaphragm of stethoscope over brachial artery.		
10.	Closes the valve (clockwise) until it stops. Does not tighten it.		

11.	Inflates cuff to between 160 mm Hg to 180 mm Hg. If beat is heard immediately upon cuff deflation, completely deflates the cuff. Reinflates cuff to no more than 200 mm Hg.		
12.	Opens the valve slightly with thumb and index finger. Deflates cuff slowly.		
13.	Watches gauge and listens for sound of pulse.		
14.	Remembers the reading at which the first pulse sound is heard. This is the systolic pressure.		
15.	Continues listening for a change or muffling of pulse sound. The point of a change or the point that the sound disappears is the diastolic pressure. Remembers this reading.		
16.	Opens the valve to deflate cuff completely. Removes cuff.		
17.	Washes hands.		
18.	Documents both systolic and diastolic pressures. Notes which arm was used.		
19.	Cleans stethoscope. Stores equipment.		
20.	Places call light within resident's reach.		

_____   _____
Date Reviewed   Instructor Signature

_____   _____
Date Performed   Instructor Signature

Applying warm compresses

	Procedure Steps	yes	no
1.	Identifies self by name. Identifies resident by name.		
2.	Washes hands.		
3.	Explains procedure to resident, speaking clearly, slowly, and directly. Maintains face-to-face contact whenever possible.		

4.	Provides privacy.		
5.	Fills basin one-half to two-thirds with warm water. Tests water temperature (no higher than 105°F). Has resident test water temperature and adjusts if necessary.		
6.	Soaks washcloth, wrings it out, and applies to area needing compress. Notes the time. Covers with plastic wrap and towel.		
7.	Checks area every five minutes. Removes compress if redness, numbness, pain, or discomfort occurs. Changes compress if cooling occurs.		
8.	Removes compress after 20 minutes.		
9.	Empties, rinses, and wipes basin and returns to storage. Places soiled towels in proper container and discards plastic wrap.		
10	Places call light within resident's reach.		
11.	Washes hands.		
12.	Documents procedure.		

_____   _____
Date Reviewed   Instructor Signature

_____   _____
Date Performed   Instructor Signature

Administering warm soaks

	Procedure Steps	yes	no
1.	Identifies self by name. Identifies resident by name.		
2.	Washes hands.		
3.	Explains procedure to resident, speaking clearly, slowly, and directly. Maintains face-to-face contact whenever possible.		
4.	Provides privacy.		

5.	Fills the basin half full of warm water. Tests water temperature (no higher than 105°F). Has resident test water temperature and adjusts if necessary.		
6.	Places basin on disposable absorbent pad, and immerses body part in water. Pads the edge of the basin as necessary. Covers resident for extra warmth if needed.		
7.	Checks water temperature every five minutes, adding hot water as needed.		
8.	Observes area for redness and discontinues soak if resident complains of pain or discomfort.		
9.	Soaks for 15 to 20 minutes or as ordered in the care plan.		
10.	Removes basin and uses a towel to dry the body part that was wet.		
11.	Empties, rinses, and wipes basin and returns to storage. Places soiled towels in proper container and discards disposable pad.		
12.	Places call light within resident's reach.		
13.	Washes hands.		
14.	Documents procedure.		

_____   _____
Date Reviewed   Instructor Signature

_____   _____
Date Performed   Instructor Signature

Applying an Aquamatic K-Pad

	Procedure Steps	yes	no
1.	Identifies self by name. Identifies resident by name.		
2.	Washes hands.		
3.	Explains procedure to resident, speaking clearly, slowly, and directly. Maintains face-to-face contact whenever possible.		

4.	Provides privacy.		
5.	Places unit on bedside table. Checks to make sure cords are not damaged and that tubing is intact.		
6.	Removes cover of control unit. Fills with distilled water to fill line if water level is low.		
7.	Puts cover of unit back on. Plugs unit in and turns pad on.		
8.	Places pad in cover.		
9.	Uncovers area to be treated. Places the pad and notes the time.		
10.	Returns to check area every five minutes, removing the pad if area is red or numb, or if resident reports pain or discomfort.		
11.	Fills with distilled water when necessary.		
12.	Removes pad after 20 minutes and turns off unit.		
13.	Cleans and stores supplies.		
14.	Places call light within resident's reach.		
15.	Washes hands.		
16.	Documents procedure.		

_____   _____
Date Reviewed   Instructor Signature

_____   _____
Date Performed   Instructor Signature

Assisting with a sitz bath

	Procedure Steps	yes	no
1.	Identifies self by name. Identifies resident by name.		
2.	Washes hands.		
3.	Explains procedure to resident, speaking clearly, slowly, and directly. Maintains face-to-face contact whenever possible.		
4.	Provides privacy.		
5.	Puts on gloves.		

6.	Fills sitz bath two-thirds full with warm water (no higher than 105°F).		
7.	Places sitz bath on toilet seat and helps resident undress and sit down on sitz bath.		
8.	Leaves the room and checks on resident every five minutes for weakness or dizziness. Stays with a resident who is unsteady.		
9.	Helps resident off of sitz bath after 20 minutes. Provides towels and helps with dressing as needed.		
10.	Cleans and stores supplies.		
11.	Removes and discards gloves.		
12.	Washes hands.		
13.	Places call light within resident's reach.		
14.	Documents procedure.		

_____   _____
Date Reviewed   Instructor Signature

_____   _____
Date Performed   Instructor Signature

Applying ice packs

	Procedure Steps	yes	no
1.	Identifies self by name. Identifies resident by name.		
2.	Washes hands.		
3.	Explains procedure to resident, speaking clearly, slowly, and directly. Maintains face-to-face contact whenever possible.		
4.	Provides privacy.		
5.	Fills plastic bag or ice pack 1/2 to 2/3 full with ice and removes excess air. Seals bag and covers bag with towel.		
6.	Applies bag to the area as ordered. Uses another towel to cover bag if it is too cold.		

7.	Notes the time and checks the area after five minutes for blisters or pale, white, or gray skin. Stops treatment if resident complains of numbness or pain.		
8.	Removes ice after 20 minutes or as ordered.		
9.	Discards or stores supplies and places towel in proper container.		
10.	Places call light within resident's reach.		
11.	Washes hands.		
12.	Documents procedure.		

_____   _____
Date Reviewed   Instructor Signature

_____   _____
Date Performed   Instructor Signature

Applying cold compresses

	Procedure Steps	yes	no
1.	Identifies self by name. Identifies resident by name.		
2.	Washes hands.		
3.	Explains procedure to resident, speaking clearly, slowly, and directly. Maintains face-to-face contact whenever possible.		
4.	Provides privacy.		
5.	Places absorbent pad under area to be treated. Rinses washcloth in basin and wrings out washcloth.		
6.	Covers the area with towel and applies cold washcloth to the area. Changes washcloths to keep area cold.		
7.	Checks the area after five minutes for blisters or pale, white, or gray skin. Stops treatment if resident complains of numbness or pain.		
8.	Removes compresses after 20 minutes or as ordered. Gives resident towels as needed to dry the area.		

9.	Discards pad. Cleans and stores basin properly. Places towels in proper container.		
10.	Places call light within resident's reach.		
11.	Washes hands.		
12.	Documents procedure.		

Date Reviewed   Instructor Signature

Date Performed   Instructor Signature

Changing a dry dressing using non-sterile technique

	Procedure Steps	yes	no
1.	Identifies self by name. Identifies resident by name.		
2.	Washes hands.		
3.	Explains procedure to resident, speaking clearly, slowly, and directly. Maintains face-to-face contact whenever possible.		
4.	Provides privacy.		
5.	Cuts pieces of tape long enough to secure the dressing. Opens gauze package without touching the gauze. Places open package on flat surface.		
6.	Puts on gloves.		
7.	Removes soiled dressing gently by peeling tape toward wound. Lifts dressing off the wound and observes dressing for odor or drainage. Notes color and size of the wound. Discards used dressing in proper container. Removes and discards gloves. Washes hands.		
8.	Puts on clean gloves.		
9.	Applies clean gauze to wound. Tapes gauze in place. Discards supplies.		
10.	Removes and discards gloves.		
11.	Washes hands.		

12.	Places call light within resident's reach.		
13.	Documents procedure.		

Date Reviewed   Instructor Signature

Date Performed   Instructor Signature

Assisting in changing clothes for a resident who has an IV

	Procedure Steps	yes	no
1.	Identifies self by name. Identifies resident by name.		
2.	Washes hands.		
3.	Explains procedure to resident, speaking clearly, slowly, and directly. Maintains face-to-face contact whenever possible.		
4.	Provides privacy.		
5.	Adjusts bed to lowest position and locks bed wheels. Helps resident to sitting position with feet flat on the floor.		
6.	Helps resident remove the arm without the IV from the clothing.		
7.	Helps resident gather clothing on arm with IV site, lifts clothing over IV site, and moves it up the tubing toward the IV bag.		
8.	Lifts IV bag off the pole, keeping it higher than the IV site, slides clothing over IV bag, and replaces IV bag on the pole.		
9.	Sets used clothing aside and gathers the sleeve of the clean clothing.		
10.	Lifts IV bag off the pole again, keeping it higher than the IV site. Slides clean clothing over IV bag onto the resident's arm, and replaces IV bag on the pole.		
11.	Moves clean clothing over tubing and IV site and onto the resident's arm.		

		yes	no
12.	Assists resident with putting other arm into clothing.		
13.	Checks the IV to make sure it is dripping. Checks the tubing and makes sure dressing is in proper place.		
14.	Assists resident with changing the rest of the clothing.		
15.	Places soiled clothes in proper container.		
16.	Places call light within resident's reach.		
17.	Washes hands.		
18.	Documents procedure.		

_____ _____
Date Reviewed   Instructor Signature

_____ _____
Date Performed   Instructor Signature

15
Nutrition and Hydration

Feeding a resident			
	Procedure Steps	yes	no
1.	Identifies self by name. Identifies resident by name.		
2.	Washes hands.		
3.	Explains procedure to resident, speaking clearly, slowly, and directly. Maintains face-to-face contact whenever possible.		
4.	Provides privacy.		
5.	Picks up diet card and asks resident to state his name. Verifies that resident has received the right tray.		
6.	Raises the head of the bed. Makes sure resident is in an upright sitting position.		
7.	Adjusts bed height to seat self at resident's eye level. Locks bed wheels.		

		yes	no
8.	Places meal tray where it can be easily seen by resident, such as on overbed table.		
9.	Helps resident clean hands if needed.		
10.	Helps resident to put on clothing protector if desired.		
11.	Sits facing resident, at resident's eye level, on resident's stronger side.		
12.	Tells resident what foods are on plate. Offers drink of beverage and asks what resident would like to eat first.		
13.	Offers the food in bite-sized pieces, telling resident content of each bite offered. Alternates types of food offered, allowing for resident's preferences. Makes sure resident's mouth is empty before next bite of food or sip of beverage.		
14.	Offers drink of beverage throughout the meal.		
15.	Talks with resident during meal.		
16.	Wipes food from resident's mouth and hands as necessary during the meal. Wipes again at the end of the meal.		
17.	Removes clothing protector if used.		
18.	Removes food tray, checking for personal items. Places tray in proper area.		
19.	Keeps resident upright for at least 30 minutes if ordered. Returns bed to lowest position.		
20.	Places call light within resident's reach.		
21.	Washes hands.		
22.	Documents procedure.		

_____ _____
Date Reviewed   Instructor Signature

_____ _____
Date Performed   Instructor Signature

Measuring and recording intake and output

	Procedure Steps	yes	no
	For measuring intake:		
1.	Identifies self by name. Identifies resident by name.		
2.	Washes hands.		
3.	Explains procedure to resident, speaking clearly, slowly, and directly. Maintains face-to-face contact whenever possible.		
4.	Provides privacy.		
5.	Notes amount of fluid resident is served and notes on paper.		
6.	Measures leftover fluid and notes on paper.		
7.	Subtracts amount left over from amount served. Converts to milliliters.		
8.	Documents amount of fluid consumed (in mL) in input column on I&O sheet. Records time and what fluid was taken.		
9.	Washes hands.		
	For measuring output:		
1.	Washes hands.		
2.	Puts on gloves.		
3.	Pours contents of bedpan or urinal into measuring container.		
4.	Measures amount of urine, keeping container level.		
5.	Discards urine without splashing. Rinses graduate and bedpan/urinal, pouring rinse water in toilet. Flushes toilet.		
6.	Places graduate and bedpan in area for cleaning or cleans and stores according to policy.		
7.	Removes and discards gloves.		
8.	Washes hands.		
9.	Documents the time and amount (in mL) of urine in output column.		

Date Reviewed _____ Instructor Signature _____

Date Performed _____ Instructor Signature _____

Serving fresh water

	Procedure Steps	yes	no
1.	Identifies self by name. Identifies resident by name.		
2.	Washes hands.		
3.	Puts on gloves.		
4.	Scoops ice into water pitcher. Adds fresh water.		
5.	Uses and stores ice scoop properly.		
6.	Takes pitcher to resident. Pours cup of water for resident and leaves pitcher and cup at bedside.		
7.	Makes sure pitcher and cup are light enough for resident to lift. Leaves a straw if resident wants one and does not have a swallowing problem.		
8.	Places call light within resident's reach.		
9.	Removes and discards gloves.		
10.	Washes hands.		

Date Reviewed _____ Instructor Signature _____

Date Performed _____ Instructor Signature _____

16
Urinary Elimination

Assisting a resident with the use of a bedpan

	Procedure Steps	yes	no
1.	Identifies self by name. Identifies resident by name.		

2.	Washes hands.		
3.	Explains procedure to resident, speaking clearly, slowly, and directly. Maintains face-to-face contact whenever possible.		
4.	Provides privacy.		
5.	Adjusts the bed to a safe level. Lowers head of bed. Locks bed wheels.		
6.	Puts on gloves.		
7.	Covers resident with bath blanket, then pulls down top covers underneath. Asks resident to remove undergarments or assists resident to do so.		
8.	Places a bed protector under resident's buttocks and hips.		
9.	Places bedpan under hips in correct position (**standard bedpan** positioned with wider end aligned with the buttocks; **fracture pan** positioned with handle toward foot of bed).		
10.	Removes and discards gloves. Washes hands.		
11.	Raises head of bed and props resident into semi-sitting position with pillows.		
12.	Makes sure blanket is covering resident. Provides resident with supplies and asks resident to clean hands with wipe when finished.		
13.	Places call light within reach and leaves room until resident calls.		
14.	When called, returns and washes hands. Puts on clean gloves. Lowers head of bed. Removes and covers bedpan.		
15.	Gives perineal care if help is needed. Assists with putting undergarments on. Covers resident and removes bath blanket. Places towel in bag and discards disposable supplies.		

16.	Takes bedpan to bathroom and empties bedpan into toilet. Rinses bedpan and empties rinse water into toilet. Flushes toilet. Places bedpan in proper area for cleaning or cleans it according to policy.		
17.	Removes and discards gloves.		
18.	Washes hands.		
19.	Returns bed to lowest position.		
20.	Places call light within resident's reach.		
21.	Documents procedure.		

_____   _____
Date Reviewed   Instructor Signature

_____   _____
Date Performed   Instructor Signature

Assisting a male resident with a urinal

	Procedure Steps	yes	no
1.	Identifies self by name. Identifies resident by name.		
2.	Washes hands.		
3.	Explains procedure to resident, speaking clearly, slowly, and directly. Maintains face-to-face contact whenever possible.		
4.	Provides privacy.		
5.	Adjusts the bed to a safe level. Locks bed wheels.		
6.	Puts on gloves.		
7.	Places bed protector under buttocks and hips.		
8.	Hands urinal to resident or places it if resident is unable. Replaces covers.		
9.	Removes and discards gloves. Washes hands.		
10.	Asks resident to clean hands with wipe when finished. Places call light within reach and leaves room until resident calls.		
11.	When called, returns and washes hands. Puts on clean gloves.		

12.	Discards wipes. Removes urinal. Discards urine and rinses urinal, emptying rinse water in toilet. Flushes toilet. Places urinal in proper area for cleaning or cleans it according to policy.		
13.	Removes and discards gloves.		
14.	Washes hands.		
15.	Returns bed to lowest position.		
16.	Places call light within resident's reach.		
17.	Documents procedure.		

_____   _____
Date Reviewed   Instructor Signature

_____   _____
Date Performed   Instructor Signature

Assisting a resident to use a portable commode or toilet

	Procedure Steps	yes	no
1.	Identifies self by name. Identifies resident by name.		
2.	Washes hands.		
3.	Explains procedure to resident, speaking clearly, slowly, and directly. Maintains face-to-face contact whenever possible.		
4.	Provides privacy.		
5.	Locks commode wheels. Locks bed wheels and makes sure resident is wearing nonskid shoes. Helps resident to bathroom or commode.		
6.	Puts on gloves.		
7.	Helps resident remove clothing and sit on toilet set. Puts toilet paper and disposable wipes within reach. Asks resident to clean hands with wipe.		
8.	Removes and discards gloves. Washes hands. Leaves room or area, leaving call light within reach.		

9.	When called, returns and washes hands. Puts on clean gloves.		
10.	Provides perineal care if help is needed. Assists with putting undergarments on. Places towel in bag and discards disposable supplies.		
11.	Removes and discards gloves. Washes hands. Helps resident back to bed.		
12.	Puts on clean gloves. Removes waste container and empties into toilet. Rinses container and empties rinse water into toilet. Flushes toilet. Places container in proper area for cleaning or cleans it according to policy.		
13.	Removes gloves and discards them.		
14.	Washes hands.		
15.	Returns bed to lowest position.		
16.	Places call light within resident's reach.		
17.	Documents procedure.		

_____   _____
Date Reviewed   Instructor Signature

_____   _____
Date Performed   Instructor Signature

Providing catheter care

	Procedure Steps	yes	no
1.	Identifies self by name. Identifies resident by name.		
2.	Washes hands.		
3.	Explains procedure to resident, speaking clearly, slowly, and directly. Maintains face-to-face contact whenever possible.		
4.	Provides privacy.		
5.	Adjusts the bed to a safe level. Locks bed wheels. Lowers head of bed and positions resident lying flat on back.		

6.	Removes or folds back top bedding, keeping resident covered with bath blanket.		
7.	Tests water temperature with thermometer or wrist. Water temperature should be no higher than 105°F. Has resident check water temperature. Adjusts if necessary.		
8.	Puts on gloves.		
9.	Places clean bed protector under buttocks.		
10.	Exposes only the area necessary to clean the catheter.		
11.	Places towel or pad under catheter tubing before washing.		
12.	Applies soap to wet washcloth and cleans area around meatus, using a clean area of the cloth for each stroke.		
13.	Holding catheter near meatus, cleans at least four inches of catheter. Moves in only one direction, away from meatus. Uses a clean area of the cloth for each stroke.		
14.	Rinses area around meatus and dries area around the meatus. Uses a clean area of the cloth for each stroke. Dries area around meatus. Rinses at least four inches of catheter nearest meatus, moving away from meatus. Dries at least four inches of catheter nearest meatus.		
15.	Removes and discards bed protector. Disposes of linen in proper containers. Empties and rinses basin. Flushes toilet. Places basin in proper area for cleaning or cleans and stores according to policy.		
16.	Removes and discards gloves.		
17.	Washes hands.		
18.	Removes bath blanket and replaces top covers.		

19.	Returns bed to lowest position.		
20.	Places call light within resident's reach.		
21.	Documents procedure.		

_____ _____
Date Reviewed   Instructor Signature

_____ _____
Date Performed   Instructor Signature

Emptying the catheter drainage bag

	Procedure Steps	yes	no
1.	Identifies self by name. Identifies resident by name.		
2.	Washes hands.		
3.	Explains procedure to resident, speaking clearly, slowly, and directly. Maintains face-to-face contact whenever possible.		
4.	Provides privacy.		
5.	Puts on gloves.		
6.	Places measuring container on paper towel on floor.		
7.	Opens clamp on drainage bag so urine flows into graduate. Does not let spout or clamp touch graduate.		
8.	Closes clamp and cleans it. Replaces drain spout in its holder on the bag.		
9.	Places graduate on flat surface in bathroom. Notes amount and appearance of urine and empties it into toilet. Flushes toilet.		
10.	Cleans and stores graduate properly. Discards paper towels.		
11.	Removes and discards gloves.		
12.	Washes hands.		
13.	Documents procedure.		

_____ _____
Date Reviewed   Instructor Signature

_____ _____
Date Performed   Instructor Signature

Changing a condom catheter

	Procedure Steps	yes	no
1.	Identifies self by name. Identifies resident by name.		
2.	Washes hands.		
3.	Explains procedure to resident, speaking clearly, slowly, and directly. Maintains face-to-face contact whenever possible.		
4.	Provides privacy.		
5.	Adjusts the bed to a safe level. Locks bed wheels. Lowers head of bed and positions resident lying flat on back.		
6.	Removes or folds back bedding, keeping resident covered with bath blanket.		
7.	Puts on gloves.		
8.	Places a clean bed protector under the buttocks. Adjusts bath blanket to expose only genital area.		
9.	Removes condom catheter if one is in place. Places condom and tape in plastic bag.		
10.	Assists as necessary with perineal care.		
11.	Moves pubic hair away from penis. Places condom on penis and rolls toward base of penis, leaving space between drainage tip and glans of penis to prevent irritation.		
12.	Gently secures a condom to penis, applying tape in a spiral manner.		
13.	Connects catheter tip to drainage tubing. Makes sure tubing is not twisted or kinked.		
14.	Discards bed protector and used supplies. Places soiled linen and clothing in proper containers. Cleans and stores supplies.		
15.	Removes and discards gloves.		
16.	Washes hands.		
17.	Returns bed to its lowest position.		
18.	Places call light within resident's reach.		
19.	Documents procedure.		

_____   _____
Date Reviewed   Instructor Signature

_____   _____
Date Performed   Instructor Signature

Collecting a routine urine specimen

	Procedure Steps	yes	no
1.	Identifies self by name. Identifies resident by name.		
2.	Washes hands.		
3.	Explains procedure to resident, speaking clearly, slowly, and directly. Maintains face-to-face contact whenever possible.		
4.	Provides privacy.		
5.	Puts on gloves.		
6.	Fits hat to toilet or commode, or offers bedpan or urinal.		
7.	Asks resident to void into hat, urinal, or bedpan. Asks resident not to put toilet paper in with the sample. Provides a plastic bag to discard toilet paper separately.		
8.	Provides resident with supplies and asks resident to clean hands with wipe when finished.		
9.	Removes and discards gloves. Washes hands.		
10.	Places call light within reach and leaves room until resident calls.		
11.	When called, returns and washes hands. Puts on clean gloves. Provides perineal care if help is needed.		
12.	Takes bedpan, urinal, or hat to the bathroom.		
13.	Pours urine into specimen container, making it at least half full.		

14.	Covers container with lid. Wipes off the outside with a paper towel and discards paper towel.		
15.	Applies label and places the container in clean specimen bag. Seals bag.		
16.	Discards extra urine. Rinses hat, urinal, or bedpan and flushes toilet. Places equipment in proper area for cleaning or cleans it according to policy.		
17.	Removes and discards gloves.		
18.	Washes hands.		
19.	Returns bed to lowest position.		
20.	Places call light within resident's reach.		
21.	Takes specimen and lab slip to proper area. Documents procedure.		

_____   _____
Date Reviewed   Instructor Signature

_____   _____
Date Performed   Instructor Signature

Collecting a clean catch (mid-stream) urine specimen

	Procedure Steps	yes	no
1.	Identifies self by name. Identifies resident by name.		
2.	Washes hands.		
3.	Explains procedure to resident, speaking clearly, slowly, and directly. Maintains face-to-face contact whenever possible.		
4.	Provides privacy.		
5.	Puts on gloves.		
6.	Opens specimen kit.		
7.	Cleans perineal area, using a clean area of wipe or clean wipe for each stroke.		
8.	Asks resident to urinate into the bedpan, urinal, or toilet, and to stop before urination is complete.		

9.	Places container under the urine stream and instructs resident to start urinating again until container is at least half full. Has resident finish urinating in bedpan, urinal, or toilet.		
10.	Assists as necessary with perineal care. Asks resident to clean his hands with a wipe.		
11.	Covers urine container with lid. Wipes off outside with a paper towel and discards paper towel.		
12.	Applies label and places the container in clean specimen bag. Seals bag.		
13.	Discards extra urine. Rinses urinal or bedpan and flushes toilet. Places equipment in proper area for cleaning or cleans it according to policy.		
14.	Removes and discards gloves.		
15.	Washes hands.		
16.	Returns bed to lowest position.		
16.	Places call light within resident's reach.		
17.	Takes specimen and lab slip to proper area. Documents procedure.		

_____   _____
Date Reviewed   Instructor Signature

_____   _____
Date Performed   Instructor Signature

Collecting a 24-hour urine specimen

	Procedure Steps	yes	no
1.	Identifies self by name. Identifies resident by name.		
2.	Washes hands.		
3.	Explains procedure to resident, speaking clearly, slowly, and directly. Maintains face-to-face contact whenever possible. Emphasizes that all urine must be saved.		
4.	Provides privacy.		

5.	Places sign on bed indicating all urine within 24 hours is being collected.		
6.	Instructs resident to completely empty the bladder. Discards urine and notes the exact time.		
7.	Labels container with resident's name, room number, date of birth, and dates and times.		
8.	Washes hands and puts on gloves each time resident voids.		
9.	Pours urine into container.		
10.	Helps with perineal care as needed. Helps resident to wash hands after each voiding.		
11.	Places equipment in proper area for cleaning or cleans it according to policy after each voiding.		
12.	Removes and discards gloves.		
13.	Washes hands.		
14.	After last void, adds urine to container. Removes sign.		
15.	Takes specimen and lab slip to proper area. Documents procedure.		

_____   _____
Date Reviewed   Instructor Signature

_____   _____
Date Performed   Instructor Signature

Testing urine with reagent strips			
	Procedure Steps	yes	no
1.	Washes hands.		
2.	Puts on gloves.		
3.	Takes strip and recaps bottle, closing bottle tightly.		
4.	Dips strip into specimen.		
5.	Removes strip at correct time.		
6.	Compares strip with color chart on bottle.		
7.	Reads results.		
8.	Stores strips. Discards used items. Discards specimen in toilet and flushes toilet.		

9.	Removes and discards gloves.		
10.	Washes hands.		
11.	Documents procedure.		

_____   _____
Date Reviewed   Instructor Signature

_____   _____
Date Performed   Instructor Signature

17
Bowel Elimination

Giving a cleansing enema			
	Procedure Steps	yes	no
1.	Identifies self by name. Identifies resident by name.		
2.	Washes hands.		
3.	Explains procedure to resident, speaking clearly, slowly, and directly. Maintains face-to-face contact whenever possible.		
4.	Provides privacy.		
5.	Adjusts bed to a safe level. Locks bed wheels.		
6.	Puts on gloves.		
7.	Places bed protector under resident. Helps remove undergarments.		
8.	Helps resident into left-sided Sims' position. Places bedpan close to resident's body. Places bedpan close to resident's body. Covers with a bath blanket.		
9.	Places IV pole beside the bed.		
10.	Clamps enema tube. Prepares enema solution. Fills bag with 500-1000 mL of warm water (105°F). Mixes solution. Checks water temperature with bath thermometer.		
11.	Unclamps tube. Lets a small amount of solution run through tubing. Re-clamps tube.		

Name: _____

12.	Hangs bag on IV pole. Makes sure bottom of bag is not more than 12 inches above the resident's anus.		
13.	Lubricates tip of tubing. Asks resident to breathe deeply.		
14.	Lifts buttock to expose anus and asks resident to take a deep breath and exhale. Gently inserts tip of tubing two to four inches into rectum.		
15.	Unclamps tubing. Allows solution to flow slowly. Encourages resident to take as much of solution as possible.		
16.	Clamps the tubing when solution is almost gone. Removes tip from rectum and places it into enema bag. Does not contaminate self, resident, or linens.		
17.	Asks the resident to hold solution inside as long as possible.		
18.	Helps resident to use bedpan, commode, or get to bathroom.		
19.	Removes and discards gloves and washes hands.		
20.	Places toilet paper or wipes within resident's reach. Asks resident to clean hands with wipes when finished.		
21.	Places call light within reach and asks resident to signal when finished. Leaves room and closes door.		
22.	When called, returns and washes hands. Puts on clean gloves. Lowers the head of the bed and removes and covers bedpan.		
23.	Helps with perineal care as needed. Helps resident put on undergarment. Covers resident and removes bath blanket.		

24.	Removes and discards bed protector. Places towel and bath blanket in a bag and discards disposable supplies. Takes bedpan to bathroom and calls nurse to observe results.		
25.	Empties and rinses bedpan. Flushes toilet. Places bedpan in proper area for cleaning or cleans it according to policy.		
26.	Removes and discards gloves.		
27.	Washes hands.		
28.	Returns bed to lowest position.		
29.	Places call light within resident's reach.		
30.	Documents procedure.		

_____ _____
Date Reviewed   Instructor Signature

_____ _____
Date Performed   Instructor Signature

Giving a commercial enema

	Procedure Steps	yes	no
1.	Identifies self by name. Identifies resident by name.		
2.	Washes hands.		
3.	Explains procedure to resident, speaking clearly, slowly, and directly. Maintains face-to-face contact whenever possible.		
4.	Provides privacy.		
5.	Adjusts bed to a safe level. Locks bed wheels.		
6.	Puts on gloves.		
7.	Places bed protector under resident. Helps remove undergarments.		
8.	Helps resident into left-sided Sims' position. Places bedpan close to resident's body. Places bedpan close to resident's body. Covers with a bath blanket.		
9.	Uncovers resident enough to expose anus only.		

10.	Lubricates tip of bottle.		
11.	Asks resident to breathe deeply during procedure.		
12.	Lifts buttock to expose anus and asks resident to take a deep breath and exhale. Gently inserts tip of tubing one and a half inches into rectum.		
13.	Slowly squeezes and rolls container so that solution runs inside the resident.		
14.	Removes tip and places bottle inside box upside down.		
15.	Asks resident to hold solution inside as long as possible.		
16.	Helps resident to use bedpan, commode, or get to bathroom.		
17.	Removes and discards gloves and washes hands.		
18.	Places toilet paper or wipes within resident's reach. Asks resident to clean hands with wipes when finished.		
19.	Places call light within reach and asks resident to signal when finished. Leaves room and closes door.		
20.	When called, returns and washes hands. Puts on clean gloves. Lowers the head of the bed and removes and covers bedpan.		
21.	Helps with perineal care as needed. Helps resident put on undergarment. Covers resident and removes bath blanket.		
22.	Removes and discards bed protector. Places towel and bath blanket in a bag and discards disposable supplies. Takes bedpan to bathroom and calls nurse to observe results.		
23.	Empties and rinses bedpan. Flushes toilet. Places bedpan in proper area for cleaning or cleans it according to policy.		
24.	Removes and discards gloves		

25.	Washes hands.		
26.	Returns bed to lowest position.		
27.	Places call light within resident's reach.		
28.	Documents procedure.		

_____   _____
Date Reviewed   Instructor Signature

_____   _____
Date Performed   Instructor Signature

Collecting a stool specimen

	Procedure Steps	yes	no
1.	Identifies self by name. Identifies resident by name.		
2.	Washes hands.		
3.	Explains procedure to resident, speaking clearly, slowly, and directly. Maintains face-to-face contact whenever possible.		
4.	Provides privacy.		
5.	Puts on gloves.		
6.	Asks resident not to urinate at the same time as moving bowels and not to put toilet paper in with the sample. Provides plastic bag to discard toilet paper separately.		
7.	Fits hat to toilet or commode, or provides resident with bedpan.		
8.	Places toilet paper or wipes within resident's reach. Asks resident to clean hands with wipes when finished.		
9.	Removes and discards gloves. Washes hands.		
10.	Places call light within reach and asks resident to signal when finished. Leaves room and closes door.		
11.	When called, returns and washes hands. Puts on clean gloves. Provides perineal care if help is needed.		

Name: _____

12.	Uses two tongue blades to take about two tablespoons of stool and puts it in container without touching the inside. Covers container tightly. Applies label and places container in clean specimen bag. Seals bag.		
13.	Discards tongue blades and toilet paper. Empties and rinses bedpan or container into toilet. Flushes toilet. Places equipment in proper area for cleaning or cleans it according to policy.		
14.	Removes and discards gloves.		
15.	Washes hands.		
16.	Places call light within resident's reach.		
17.	Takes specimen and lab slip to proper area. Documents procedure.		

_____   _____
Date Reviewed   Instructor Signature

_____   _____
Date Performed   Instructor Signature

9.	Waits the proper amount of time. Watches squares for color changes and records any changes.		
10.	Places tongue blade and test packet in plastic bag. Disposes of plastic bag properly.		
11.	Removes and discards gloves.		
12.	Washes hands.		
13.	Documents procedure.		

_____   _____
Date Reviewed   Instructor Signature

_____   _____
Date Performed   Instructor Signature

Testing a stool specimen for occult blood

	Procedure Steps	yes	no
1.	Washes hands.		
2.	Puts on gloves.		
3.	Opens test card.		
4.	Gets small amount of stool from specimen container with tongue blade.		
5.	Smears small amount of stool onto Box A of test card.		
6.	Flips tongue blade and gets some stool from another part of specimen. Smears small amount of stool onto Box B of test card.		
7.	Closes test card and turns over to other side.		
8.	Opens the flap and opens developer. Applies developer to each box.		

Caring for an ostomy

	Procedure Steps	yes	no
1.	Identifies self by name. Identifies resident by name.		
2.	Washes hands.		
3.	Explains procedure to resident, speaking clearly, slowly, and directly. Maintains face-to-face contact whenever possible.		
4.	Provides privacy.		
5.	Adjusts the bed to a safe level. Locks bed wheels.		
6.	Puts on gloves.		
7.	Places bed protector under resident. Covers resident with a bath blanket and only exposes the ostomy site. Offers resident a towel.		
8.	Removes ostomy pouch carefully and places it in plastic bag. Notes color, odor, consistency, and amount of stool in the bag.		
9.	Wipes area around the stoma with wipes. Discards wipes in plastic bag.		

		yes	no
10.	Washes area around the stoma using a washcloth and warm, soapy water. Moves in one direction, away from the stoma. Rinses and pats dry with another towel.		
11.	Places the clean ostomy drainage pouch on resident. Holds in place and seals securely. Makes sure the bottom of the pouch is clamped.		
12.	Removes and discards bed protector. Places soiled linens in proper container. Discards plastic bag.		
13.	Removes and discards gloves.		
14.	Washes hands.		
15.	Returns bed to lowest position.		
16.	Places call light within resident's reach.		
17.	Documents procedure.		

_____   _____
Date Reviewed   Instructor Signature

_____   _____
Date Performed   Instructor Signature

18
Common Chronic and Acute Conditions

Putting elastic stockings on a resident			
	Procedure Steps	yes	no
1.	Identifies self by name. Identifies resident by name.		
2.	Washes hands.		
3.	Explains procedure to resident, speaking clearly, slowly, and directly. Maintains face-to-face contact whenever possible.		
4.	Provides privacy.		
5.	With resident in supine position, removes his socks, shoes, or slippers, and exposes one leg.		
6.	Turns stocking inside out at least to heel area.		

		yes	no
7.	Gently places the foot of the stocking over toes, foot, and heel. Heel should be in right place (heel of foot should be in heel of stocking).		
8.	Gently pulls top of stocking over foot, heel, and leg.		
9.	Makes sure that there are no twists and wrinkles in the stocking after it is applied.		
10.	Repeats for the other leg.		
11.	Places call light within resident's reach.		
12.	Washes hands.		
13.	Documents procedure.		

_____   _____
Date Reviewed   Instructor Signature

_____   _____
Date Performed   Instructor Signature

Collecting a sputum specimen			
	Procedure Steps	yes	no
1.	Identifies self by name. Identifies resident by name.		
2.	Washes hands.		
3.	Explains procedure to resident, speaking clearly, slowly, and directly. Maintains face-to-face contact whenever possible.		
4.	Provides privacy.		
5.	Puts on mask and gloves. Stands behind the resident if resident can hold container by himself.		
6.	Gives resident tissues to cover the mouth. Asks resident to cough deeply and spit the sputum into the container.		
7.	After sample has been obtained, covers container tightly, and wipes any sputum off the outside of the container. Applies label and puts container in clean specimen bag. Seals bag.		

Name: _____

8.	Removes and discards gloves and mask.		
9.	Washes hands.		
10.	Places call light within resident's reach.		
11.	Documents procedure.		

_____ _____
Date Reviewed   Instructor Signature

_____ _____
Date Performed   Instructor Signature

Providing foot care for a resident with diabetes

	Procedure Steps	yes	no
1.	Identifies self by name. Identifies resident by name.		
2.	Washes hands.		
3.	Explains procedure to resident, speaking clearly, slowly, and directly. Maintains face-to-face contact whenever possible.		
4.	Provides privacy.		
5.	Fills basin halfway with warm water. Tests water temperature (no higher than 105°F). Has resident test water temperature and adjusts if necessary.		
6.	Places basin at comfortable position. Puts on gloves.		
7.	Completely submerges feet in water and soaks feet for 10 to 20 minutes, adding warm water as necessary.		
8.	Washes feet with washcloth and soap and rinses in warm water.		
9.	Pats the feet dry, wiping between the toes.		
10.	Gently rubs lotion into the feet with circular strokes. Does not put lotion between the toes.		
11.	Observes the skin for signs of dryness, irritation, blisters, redness, sores, corns, discoloration, or swelling.		

12.	Helps resident with putting on socks and shoes or slippers.		
13.	Empties, rinses, and dries basin. Places basin in designated area or returns to storage, and places soiled clothing and linens in proper containers.		
14.	Removes and discards gloves and washes hands.		
15.	Places call light within resident's reach.		
16.	Documents procedure.		

_____ _____
Date Reviewed   Instructor Signature

_____ _____
Date Performed   Instructor Signature

21
Rehabilitation and Restorative Care

Assisting with passive range of motion exercises

	Procedure Steps	yes	no
1.	Identifies self by name. Identifies resident by name.		
2.	Washes hands.		
3.	Explains procedure to resident, speaking clearly, slowly, and directly. Maintains face-to-face contact whenever possible.		
4.	Provides privacy.		
5.	Adjusts the bed to a safe level. Locks bed wheels.		
6.	Positions resident in supine position.		
7.	Repeats each exercise at least three times.		
8.	**Shoulder:** Performs the following movements properly, supporting the resident's arm at the elbow and wrist by placing one hand under the elbow and the other hand under the wrist:		

Name: _____

1. Extension		
2. Flexion		
3. Abduction		
4. Adduction		
Elbow: Performs the following movements properly, holding the wrist with one hand, and holding the elbow with the other:		
1. Flexion		
2. Extension		
3. Pronation		
4. Supination		
Wrist: Performs the following movements properly, holding the wrist with one hand and using the fingers of the other hand to help the joint through the motions:		
1. Flexion		
2. Dorsiflexion		
3. Radial flexion		
4. Ulnar flexion		
Thumb: Performs the following movements properly:		
1. Abduction		
2. Adduction		
3. Opposition		
4. Flexion		
5. Extension		
Fingers: Performs the following movements properly:		
1. Flexion		
2. Extension		
3. Abduction		
4. Adduction		

	Hip: Performs the following movements properly, placing one hand under the knee and one under the ankle:		
	1. Abduction		
	2. Adduction		
	3. Internal rotation		
	4. External rotation		
	Knees: Performs the following movements properly, placing one hand under the knee and one under the ankle:		
	1. Flexion		
	2. Extension		
	Ankles: Performs the following movements properly, supporting the foot and ankle:		
	1. Dorsiflexion		
	2. Plantar flexion		
	3. Supination		
	4. Pronation		
	Toes: Performs the following movements properly:		
	1. Flexion		
	2. Extension		
	3. Abduction		
	When all exercises are completed:		
9.	Returns resident to comfortable position and covers as appropriate. Returns bed to lowest position.		
10.	Places call light within resident's reach.		
11.	Washes hands.		

12.	Documents procedure. Notes any decrease in range of motion or any pain experienced by the resident. Notifies nurse if increased stiffness or physical resistance is noted.		

_____ _____
Date Reviewed   Instructor Signature

_____ _____
Date Performed   Instructor Signature

25
Infection Prevention and Safety in the Home

Disinfecting using wet heat			
	Procedure Steps	yes	no
1.	Washes hands.		
2.	Places items in the pot and fills it with water, covering all items.		
3.	Places lid on pot and places pot on stove.		
4.	Turns on heat and brings water to a boil. Boils for 20 minutes.		
5.	Turns off heat. Allows items and water to cool.		
6.	After items have cooled, removes cover and then items. Places items on rack or towel to dry.		
7.	Washes and dries equipment. Returns to proper storage.		
8.	Washes hands.		
9.	Documents procedure.		

_____ _____
Date Reviewed   Instructor Signature

_____ _____
Date Performed   Instructor Signature

Disinfecting using dry heat			
	Procedure Steps	yes	no
1.	Washes hands.		
2.	Places items in the pan and places pan or sheet in oven.		

3.	Turns on oven to 350°F and bakes for one hour.		
4.	Turns off heat. Allows items to cool.		
5.	After items have cooled, removes items.		
6.	Stores items.		
7.	Washes and dries equipment. Returns to proper storage.		
8.	Washes hands.		
9.	Documents procedure.		

_____ _____
Date Reviewed   Instructor Signature

_____ _____
Date Performed   Instructor Signature

27
New Mothers, Infants, and Children

Picking up and holding a baby			
	Procedure Steps	yes	no
1.	Washes hands.		
2.	Supports the head at all times when lifting or holding the baby. With the other hand, supports the baby's back and bottom.		
3.	Performs cradle hold properly.		
4.	Performs football hold properly.		
5.	Performs upright hold properly.		

_____ _____
Date Reviewed   Instructor Signature

_____ _____
Date Performed   Instructor Signature

Sterilizing bottles			
	Procedure Steps	yes	no
1.	Washes hands.		
2.	Boils water and puts equipment in pot.		
3.	Re-boils water for five minutes.		
4.	Removes equipment with tongs and puts it on clean towels. Stores when dry.		

5.	Discards water in pot.		

Date Reviewed	Instructor Signature

Date Performed	Instructor Signature

Assisting with bottle feeding

	Procedure Steps	yes	no
1.	Washes hands.		
2.	Prepares bottle.		
3.	Sits and holds baby properly.		
4.	Inserts bottle nipple into baby's mouth, and ensures that baby's head is higher than body.		
5.	Talks or sings to baby during feeding.		
6.	Burps baby, changes diaper, and puts baby down.		
7.	Washes hands. Documents feeding.		
8.	Discards unused formula. Washes bottle, nipple, and ring and allows to air dry. Sterilizes before next use.		

Date Reviewed	Instructor Signature

Date Performed	Instructor Signature

Burping a baby

	Procedure Steps	yes	no
1.	Washes hands.		
2.	Picks baby up, using either of the two safe positions. Places burp cloth under baby's chin.		
3.	Pats back gently until baby burps.		
4.	Returns baby to safe position.		

Date Reviewed	Instructor Signature

Date Performed	Instructor Signature

Giving an infant sponge bath

	Procedure Steps	yes	no
1.	Washes hands.		
2.	Puts on gloves.		
3.	Pads the surface that baby will lie on. Fills basin and tests temperature.		
4.	Holds baby in football hold and washes eyes, then rest of face, using no soap.		
5.	Holds baby in football hold and washes hair.		
6.	Lays baby down, keeping one hand on baby.		
7.	Undresses upper body and washes it. Dries and covers the baby.		
8.	Undresses lower body and washes and dries it.		
9.	Washes perineal area properly.		
10.	Washes bottom and dries completely.		
11.	Applies lotion, keeping baby covered.		
12.	Diapers and dresses baby. Returns baby to safe position.		
13.	Discards water, cleans supplies, and discards gloves.		
14.	Washes hands.		
15.	Documents procedure.		

Date Reviewed	Instructor Signature

Date Performed	Instructor Signature

Giving an infant tub bath

	Procedure Steps	yes	no
1.	Washes hands.		
2.	Puts on gloves.		
3.	Pads the surface that baby will lie on. Fills basin and tests temperature.		

Name: _____

4.	Holds baby in football hold and washes eyes, then rest of face, using no soap.		
5.	Holds baby in football hold and washes hair.		
6.	Lays baby down, undresses, and immerses baby in basin, keeping head above water.		
7.	Uses washcloth to wash from neck down.		
8.	Removes from bath and covers immediately.		
9.	Applies lotion, keeping baby covered.		
10.	Diapers and dresses baby. Returns baby to safe position.		
11.	Discards water, cleans supplies, and discards gloves.		
12.	Washes hands.		
13.	Documents procedure.		

_____   _____
Date Reviewed   Instructor Signature

_____   _____
Date Performed   Instructor Signature

Changing cloth or disposable diapers

	Procedure Steps	yes	no
1.	Washes hands.		
2.	Puts on gloves.		
3.	Undresses baby as necessary and removes soiled diaper.		
4.	Cleans perineal area.		
5.	Allows air to circulate and applies ointment as necessary.		
6.	Applies clean cloth or disposable diaper properly.		
7.	Dresses baby and returns to safe position.		
8.	Disposes of soiled diaper.		
9.	Removes and discards gloves.		
10.	Washes hands.		
11.	Cleans area and stores supplies.		

12.	Washes hands again as needed.		
13.	Documents procedure.		

_____   _____
Date Reviewed   Instructor Signature

_____   _____
Date Performed   Instructor Signature

Measuring a baby's weight

	Procedure Steps	yes	no
1.	Washes hands.		
2.	Places infant scale on firm surface.		
3.	Places clean paper or pad on scale.		
4.	Starts with scale balanced at zero. Undresses baby.		
5.	Places baby on scale, keeping at least one hand on the baby at all times.		
6.	Reads and remembers weight.		
7.	Removes and dresses baby. Puts baby down safely.		
8.	Washes hands.		
9.	Documents weight.		

_____   _____
Date Reviewed   Instructor Signature

_____   _____
Date Performed   Instructor Signature

Measuring a baby's length

	Procedure Steps	yes	no
1.	Washes hands.		
2.	Prepares firm surface with clean sheet with inch markings. Places baby on firm surface, keeping one hand on baby at all times.		
3.	Places baby's head at beginning of measured markings. Straightens baby's knee.		
4.	Makes pencil mark on paper at baby's heel.		

5.	Determines and remembers length.		
6.	Removes baby and puts baby down safely.		
7.	Washes hands.		
8.	Documents the length.		
	When a paper with inch markings is not available:		
1.	Washes hands.		
2.	Prepares firm surface with clean sheet of paper. Places baby on firm surface, keeping one hand on baby at all times.		
3.	Makes pencil mark on paper at top of baby's head.		
4.	Straightens baby's knee.		
5.	Makes another mark at baby's heel.		
6.	Removes baby and puts baby down safely.		
7.	With tape measure, measures and remembers distance between marks.		
8.	Washes hands.		
9.	Documents length.		

_____   _____
Date Reviewed   Instructor Signature

_____   _____
Date Performed   Instructor Signature

Taking an infant's axillary, tympanic, or temporal artery temperature

	Procedure Steps	yes	no
1.	Washes hands.		
2.	Prepares thermometer.		
3.	**For axillary temperature:** Undresses baby on one side and lays baby down. Takes temperature, keeping thermometer in place for three to five minutes or until signal sounds.		

	For tympanic temperature: Lays baby on side. Takes temperature, making sure ear is sealed, until signal sounds.		
	For temporal artery temperature: Places thermometer flat on the forehead, while pressing and holding scan button. Gently sweeps thermometer across the baby's forehead, keeping thermometer intact with the skin. Releases scan button.		
4.	For all methods, removes thermometer and reads temperature. Dresses baby and puts down safely.		
5.	Cleans and stores thermometer.		
6.	Washes hands.		
7.	Documents temperature.		

_____   _____
Date Reviewed   Instructor Signature

_____   _____
Date Performed   Instructor Signature

29
The Clean, Safe, and Healthy Home Environment

Cleaning a bathroom

	Procedure Steps	yes	no
1.	Puts on gloves.		
2.	Wipes all surfaces with disinfectant and rag/wipe.		
3.	Wipes toilet bowl, using different rag.		
4.	Cleans bathtub, shower, and sink, using a different rag.		
5.	Scrubs inside of toilet bowl with brush.		
6.	Washes floor.		
7.	Cleans mirror and all glass.		
8.	Disposes of soiled towels and waste.		
9.	Stores supplies. Removes and discards gloves.		

| 10. | Washes hands. | | |
| 11. | Documents procedure. | | |

_____   _____
Date Reviewed   Instructor Signature

_____   _____
Date Performed   Instructor Signature

Doing the laundry

	Procedure Steps	yes	no
1.	Sorts clothes carefully, checking pockets and garments.		
2.	Pretreats clothes as necessary.		
3.	Uses correct temperature, laundry products, and washing cycle.		
4.	Dries clothes.		
5.	Hand washes items as necessary.		
6.	Folds and hangs clean laundry. Stores clothes.		

_____   _____
Date Reviewed   Instructor Signature

_____   _____
Date Performed   Instructor Signature

Practice Exam

Taking an Exam

After a nursing assistant has completed an approved training program in his or her state, he or she is given a competency evaluation (a certification exam or test) in order to be certified to work in that state. This exam usually consists of both a written evaluation and a skills evaluation. Here are some guidelines for taking exams to help you feel better prepared.

Your physical condition affects your mental abilities. Before taking an exam, get plenty of sleep and watch what you eat and drink. On the day of the exam, eat a healthy breakfast. It can be hard to think if you are hungry or if you did not eat a balanced breakfast. Avoid foods that contain simple sugars like soda and doughnuts.

Being in good physical shape allows for more blood to get to the brain. If you get regular physical exercise, your body will use oxygen more effectively than it would if you were out of shape. Even exercising a few days before an exam can make a noticeable difference in thinking abilities.

When taking the exam, listen carefully to any instructions given. Be sure to read the directions. When taking a multiple-choice test, first eliminate answers you know are wrong. Since your first choice is usually correct, do not change your answers unless you are sure of the correction.

Do not spend too much time on any one question. If you do not understand it, move on and go back if time allows. When you are finished with the test, review your answers. For the skills portion of the exam, review the procedures in the book and any notes you may have taken from lectures.

Many testing companies have information available on their websites regarding how to reschedule exams, supplies needed for a particular skill, what to bring to the testing site, and what to wear on the day of the exam. You will need to know who performs the testing for your state.

Some of the testing sites are listed below. Their websites have more information about the testing process.

- Pearson VUE (pearsonvue.com)

- D&S Diversified Technologies/Headmaster (hdmaster.com)

- Prometric (prometric.com)

Remember that being nervous is natural. Most people get nervous before and during a test. A little stress can actually help you focus and make you more alert. A few deep breaths can help calm you down. Try it. Most importantly, believe in yourself. You can do it!

Practice Exam

1. When a resident refuses to let the nursing assistant take her blood pressure, the nursing assistant should
    (A) Let the resident know that she must have it taken to prevent a serious illness
    (B) Take the resident's blood pressure anyway and agree to report the refusal later
    (C) Promise the resident a gift if she allows her blood pressure to be measured
    (D) Report this to the nurse

2. One task commonly assigned to nursing assistants is
    (A) Inserting and removing tubes
    (B) Changing sterile dressings
    (C) Helping residents with elimination needs
    (D) Prescribing medications to residents

3. A nursing assistant may share a resident's medical information with which of the following?
    (A) The resident's family
    (B) Other members of the healthcare team
    (C) The nursing assistant's family
    (D) The resident's roommate

4. To best communicate with a resident who has a hearing impairment, the nursing assistant should
   (A) Use short sentences and simple words
   (B) Shout the words slowly
   (C) Approach the resident from behind
   (D) Raise the pitch of her voice

5. If a nursing assistant suspects that a resident is being abused, she should
   (A) Ask the resident if he thinks he is being abused
   (B) Call the resident's family immediately to report the possible abuse
   (C) Report it to the nurse immediately
   (D) Check with the resident's roommate to see if he has noticed anything

6. An ombudsman is a person who
   (A) Is in charge of hiring facility staff
   (B) Teaches nursing assistants how to perform range of motion exercises
   (C) Is a legal advocate for residents and helps protect their rights
   (D) Creates special diets for residents who are ill

7. To best respond to a resident with Alzheimer's disease who is repeating a question over and over again, the nursing assistant should
   (A) Answer questions each time they are asked, using the same words
   (B) Try to silence the resident
   (C) Ask the resident to stop repeating herself
   (D) Explain to the resident that she just asked that question

8. With regard to a resident's toenails, a nursing assistant should
   (A) Never cut them
   (B) Cut them when the resident requests it
   (C) Cut them weekly
   (D) File them into rounded edges

9. When providing personal care, the nursing assistant should
   (A) Make sure the resident remains silent
   (B) Provide privacy for the resident
   (C) Tell the resident about other residents' conditions to distract him
   (D) Discuss her personal problems

10. Generally speaking, the last sense to leave a dying person is the sense of
    (A) Sight
    (B) Taste
    (C) Smell
    (D) Hearing

11. Which temperature site is considered the most accurate?
    (A) Rectum (rectal)
    (B) Mouth (oral)
    (C) Armpit (axilla)
    (D) Ear (tympanic)

12. How should a standard bedpan be positioned?
    (A) It should be positioned however the resident prefers.
    (B) The wider end should be aligned with the resident's buttocks.
    (C) The smaller end should be aligned with the resident's buttocks.
    (D) The smaller end should be facing the resident's head.

13. A resident tells a nursing assistant that she is scared of dying. Which would be the best response by the nursing assistant?
    (A) The NA can offer to call her minister to see if he can visit the resident.
    (B) The NA can listen quietly and ask questions when appropriate.
    (C) The NA can reassure the resident that she is not dying soon.
    (D) The NA can suggest other medications that might help with the resident's condition.

14. To prevent dehydration, a nursing assistant should
    (A) Discourage fluids before bedtime
    (B) Withhold fluids so the resident will be really thirsty
    (C) Offer fresh water and other fluids often
    (D) Wake the resident during the night to offer fluids

15. When giving perineal care to a female resident, a nursing assistant should
    (A) Wipe from front to back
    (B) Wipe from back to front
    (C) Use the same section of the washcloth for cleaning each part
    (D) Wash the anal area before the perineal area

16. If a nursing assistant sees a resident masturbating, the nursing assistant should
    (A) Ask the charge nurse what she is legally allowed to do
    (B) Provide privacy for the resident
    (C) Suggest that nighttime might be better for masturbating
    (D) Ask the resident to stop masturbating

17. In what order should range of motion exercises be performed?
    (A) Start from the feet and work up
    (B) Start from the shoulders and work down
    (C) The arms and legs should be exercised first
    (D) The arms and legs should be exercised last

18. A nursing assistant must wear gloves when
    (A) Combing a resident's hair
    (B) Feeding a resident
    (C) Performing oral care
    (D) Performing range of motion exercises

19. To best communicate with a resident who has a vision impairment, the nursing assistant should
    (A) Rearrange furniture without telling the resident
    (B) Identify herself when she enters the room
    (C) Keep the lighting low at all times
    (D) Touch the resident before identifying herself

20. The first stage of a pressure injury may have skin that is this color:
    (A) Black
    (B) Freckled
    (C) Red
    (D) Blue

21. Which one of the following statements is generally true of the normal aging process and late adulthood (65 years and older)?
    (A) People become helpless and lonely.
    (B) People become incontinent.
    (C) People develop Alzheimer's disease.
    (D) People remain active and engaged.

22. Abdominal thrusts help
    (A) Stop bleeding
    (B) Remove blockage from an airway
    (C) Reduce the risk of falls
    (D) Stop a heart attack

23. Which of the following is a way to prevent unintended weight loss?
    (A) Insisting that residents eat whatever food is offered to them
    (B) Asking residents to swallow more quickly
    (C) Offering gifts to residents who complete their meals
    (D) Honoring food likes and dislikes

24. Which of the following is a way for a nursing assistant to use proper body mechanics while working?
    (A) Bending his knees while lifting
    (B) Standing with his feet close together while lifting
    (C) Holding objects far away from his body when carrying them
    (D) Twisting at the waist when he is moving an object

25. What would be the best way for a nursing assistant to promote a resident's independence and dignity during bowel or bladder retraining?
    (A) Rushing the resident during elimination
    (B) Providing privacy for elimination
    (C) Criticizing a resident when he has a setback to help keep him motivated
    (D) Withholding fluids when the resident is incontinent

26. A resident tells a nursing assistant that he wants to wear his gray sweater. The nursing assistant should
    (A) Tell him that she has already picked out his clothes for the day
    (B) Assist him in getting dressed in his gray sweater
    (C) Tell him that his gray sweater does not match his pants and ask him to pick something else
    (D) Tell him that she likes his blue sweater better

27. When donning personal protective equipment (PPE), which of the following should be put on first?
    (A) Mask
    (B) Gown
    (C) Gloves
    (D) Goggles

28. How should soiled bed linens be handled?
    (A) By carrying them away from the nursing assistant's body
    (B) By shaking them in the air to get rid of contaminants
    (C) By taking them into another resident's room to put them in a hamper
    (D) By rolling them dirty side out

29. What is the purpose of the Health Insurance Portability and Accountability Act (HIPAA)?
    (A) To monitor quality of care in facilities
    (B) To reduce incidents of abuse in facilities
    (C) To keep protected health information private and secure
    (D) To provide training for facility staff

30. One safety device that helps transfer residents is called a
    (A) Waist restraint
    (B) Posey vest
    (C) Transfer belt
    (D) Geriatric chair

31. At which site is body temperature measured via the forehead?
    (A) Axilla
    (B) Tympanic
    (C) Temporal artery
    (D) Rectal

32. A nursing assistant should encourage a resident's independence and self-care because doing this
    (A) Promotes body function
    (B) Decreases blood flow
    (C) Lowers self-esteem
    (D) Increases anxiety

33. A restraint can be applied
    (A) When a resident is being rude to staff
    (B) When a nursing assistant does not have time to watch the resident
    (C) With a doctor's order
    (D) When a resident keeps pressing his call light

34. A nursing assistant can show she is listening carefully to a resident by
    (A) Looking away when the resident talks
    (B) Changing the subject often
    (C) Interrupting the resident to finish what he is saying
    (D) Focusing on the resident and giving feedback

35. How many milliliters equal one ounce?
    (A) 40
    (B) 30
    (C) 60
    (D) 20

36. With urinary catheters, it is important for a nursing assistant to remember that
    (A) Tubing should remain kinked and clean
    (B) Perineal care does not need to be performed
    (C) The drainage bag should be kept lower than the hips or the bladder
    (D) The tubing should be placed underneath the resident's body

37. When assisting a resident who has had a stroke, a nursing assistant should
    (A) Do everything for the resident
    (B) Lead with the stronger side when transferring
    (C) Dress the stronger side first
    (D) Place food in the weaker side of the mouth

38. In which stage would a dying resident be if he insists that a mistake was made on his blood test and he is not really dying?
    (A) Denial
    (B) Bargaining
    (C) Acceptance
    (D) Depression

39. The process of helping to restore a person to the highest level of functioning is called
    (A) Positioning
    (B) Rehabilitation
    (C) Elimination
    (D) Retention

40. A nursing assistant overhears other nursing assistants discussing a resident. One of them says that she does not like taking care of this resident because "he is rude and smells funny." The nursing assistant should
    (A) Join in the conversation and tell the others her opinion of this resident
    (B) Let the resident know so that he will be nicer to the nursing assistants
    (C) Suggest to the nursing assistants that this is not the place to have this discussion
    (D) Ask another resident's opinion about how she should respond

41. An oral temperature should not be taken on a resident who has eaten or had fluids in the last _____ minutes.
    (A) 25-35
    (B) 10-20
    (C) 40-50
    (D) 50-60

42. How many feet does a quad cane have?
    (A) 1
    (B) 2
    (C) 3
    (D) 4

43. A nursing assistant can assist residents with their spiritual needs by
    (A) Trying to convince residents to change to the nursing assistant's religion
    (B) Listening to residents talk about their beliefs
    (C) Insisting residents participate in religious services
    (D) Expressing judgments about residents' religious groups

44. When may a nursing assistant hit a resident?
    (A) When the resident becomes combative
    (B) When the resident threatens to hit the nursing assistant or someone else
    (C) Only if the resident hits the nursing assistant first
    (D) Never

45. When a resident has right-sided weakness, how should clothing be applied first?
    (A) On the left side
    (B) On the right side
    (C) On whichever side is closer to the nursing assistant
    (D) On whichever side the resident prefers

46. A resident offers a nursing assistant a gift for being such a good nursing assistant. The nursing assistant should
    (A) Politely refuse the gift
    (B) Politely accept the gift
    (C) Accept the gift but donate it
    (D) Ask the resident for money instead

47. According to OBRA, nursing assistants must complete at least ___ hours of training and must pass a competency evaluation before they can be employed.
    (A) 100
    (B) 250
    (C) 50
    (D) 75

48. Call lights should be placed
    (A) High on the wall over the head of the bed
    (B) Inside the bedside stand
    (C) On the floor
    (D) Within the resident's reach

49. How long should nursing assistants use friction when lathering and washing their hands?
    (A) 2 minutes
    (B) 5 seconds
    (C) 18 seconds
    (D) 20 seconds

50. The Occupational Safety and Health Administration (OSHA) is a federal government agency that protects workers from
    (A) Hazards on the job
    (B) Lawsuits
    (C) Workplace violence
    (D) Unfair employment practices